BEATING
ADHD
NATURALLY

Dr. Scott A. Johnson

Cover design: Scott A. Johnson
Cover copyright: Scott A. Johnson © 2016

Beating ADHD Naturally/Scott A. Johnson

ISBN-13: 978-0996413978

ISBN-10: 0996413979

Published by Scott A. Johnson Professional Writing Services, LLC

Printed by Create Space, an Amazon.com company

Discover more books by Scott A. Johnson at authorscott.com

DEDICATION

To my wife—who is the best friend I have in this world—and children—who inspire me and bring me joy:

Your willing sacrifices that permit me to help others across the globe discover greater wellness do not go unacknowledged or unappreciated. You are the foremost reason I passionately research, write, and teach. I do so in hopes that I will raise a healthier generation that enjoys life to the fullest, and has a diminished disease burden by relying on the plentiful blessings provided by our Creator.

- Scott A. Johnson

Contents

1

The ADHD Outbreak

We are witnessing a skyrocketing prevalence of attention deficit and hyperactivity disorder (also known as hyperkinetic disorder) that has catapulted ADHD to a global quandary. Approximately 11 percent of children in the United States aged four to seventeen have been diagnosed with ADHD as of 2011.[1] That represents millions of children—not to mention the adults—who are reliant upon stimulant medications to perform at school and function in everyday situations that those who don't have ADHD don't think twice about. But a growing number of experts suggest that ADHD has become the most prevalent childhood psychiatric disorder, not necessarily because more children have the disorder, but because multiple factors are leading children and adults to be diagnosed despite insufficient symptoms. As an ever-increasing number of fidgety children and careless and impatient adults are being diagnosed and prescribed medication, now is the time to take steps to reverse the trend and *Beat ADHD Naturally.*

One of the most common childhood disorders today, ADHD can continue through adolescence and adulthood. Boys are about three times more likely to be diagnosed with ADHD than girls—a fact scientists don't fully understand. It is usually diagnosed during early school years when teachers or a parent recognize a child has difficulty paying attention. The well-recognized and classic symptoms of ADHD include difficulty focusing or paying attention, behavioral challenges, impulsivity, and hyperactivity. While these are normal behaviors witnessed in all children, children with ADHD exhibit them more frequently, or they are more severe and impair the person's ability to function socially, academically, and domestically.

History of ADHD

Modern research and technology have linked ADHD to deficits in the functioning of several areas of the brain—prefrontal cortex, the basal ganglia, parietal cortex, cerebellum, and temporal cortex. These areas of the brain are vital to memory, inhibitions, planning and organization, motivation, processing speed, attention, and impulsivity. This technology was not available in the past, which may be one factor explaining why diagnoses are increasing so dramatically. Instead, early physicians had to rely on the symptoms manifested alone.

The first mention of an attention deficit disorder occurred in 1902 when British pediatrician Sir George Still found that some children could not control their behavior despite normal intelligence. He described it as "an abnormal defect of moral control in children." Then in 1936, the US Food and Drug Administration approved Benzedrine as a nasal and bronchial decongestant. Not too long after its release, people reported it had a significant energizing side effect. Dr. Charles Bradley noticed the energizing side effect of this new medicine and further discovered that it improved school and behavioral performance in young children. Eventually, scientists, mathematicians, poets, and novelists all jumped on the Benzedrine bandwagon, using it habitually to enhance performance and productivity.

This popular practice of using "bennies" to maintain a strenuous work discipline began to fall out of favor when people noticed that it ruined their bodies when taken routinely. Benzedrine became a prescription drug in 1959, but by then the benny fad was plummeting. This decline in Benzedrine use led to the development of other drugs. The psychostimulant Ritalin (methylphenidate) was introduced in 1955 for lethargy, depression, disturbed senile behavior, psychoses and psychoneuroses associated with depression, and narcolepsy.[2] Later, in 1961, it was used for ADHD and quickly became the drug of choice for ADHD treatment. Its use as an ADHD treatment steadily increased in the 1970s until its use exploded in the 1990s—increasing 500 percent from 1991 to 1999 alone. However, ADHD wasn't officially recognized as a disorder until the release of the second edition of the DSM in 1968 (called hyperkinetic impulse disorder).

The ADHD Diagnosis Outbreak

As scientists continue to learn more about ADHD, some in the lay public dismiss it as nothing more than a fictional disorder with no biological basis, or chalk it up to poor parenting. However, compelling evidence suggests that it has a genetic and biological origin. In 2009 and 2010, scientists discovered that the traits of ADHD were highly inheritable (genetic).[3,4] Moreover, numerous brain-imaging studies have found that there are distinct differences between the brains of people with and without ADHD. What scientists have observed is that people with ADHD have fewer dopamine receptors in specific regions of the brain—a condition that would impair normal brain function and alter mood and behavior.[5,6,7] While some children may be diagnosed out of convenience or a desire to explain troublesome behavior, it is clear that ADHD has a psychophysiological basis.

Diagnosing children with the neurobehavioral disorder ADHD has rapidly increased over the last few decades. Only one in twenty (5 percent) US children were diagnosed with ADHD during the 1980s. That number has progressively increased to more than one in ten, or 6.4 million children in the United States by 2011.[8] From 1996 to 2006 the rates of ADHD diagnosis increased an average of 3 percent per year.[9] Interestingly, boys are four times more likely to be diagnosed with ADHD than girls. It is possible that girls are diagnosed less frequently because they are more likely than boys to have the inattentive form of ADHD, the symptoms of which are not as obvious as the hyperactive-impulsive subtypes of ADHD. Indeed, adult women tend to self-refer for ADHD as they begin to see common behaviors between their children and themselves.

Although ADHD is considered a childhood disease that one can grow out of during adulthood, it is now evident that ADHD persists in up to 66 percent of adults.[10,11,12,13] It is estimated that just over 4 percent of the adult population suffers from ADHD (range 1.2%–7.3%).[14,15] The challenges of ADHD in adulthood can be more problematic, because difficulty following directions, concentrating, organizing, managing time, and remembering information can disrupt school, work, and personal life. Adults with ADHD are more likely to change jobs frequently, perform poorly, and be less satisfied with their jobs. In addition, adults with ADHD experience more marital problems, are more likely to engage in risky behaviors (smoking, alcohol, and drug use), get more speeding tickets, and are less financially stable. The significant problems associated with adult ADHD often require and improve with treatment.

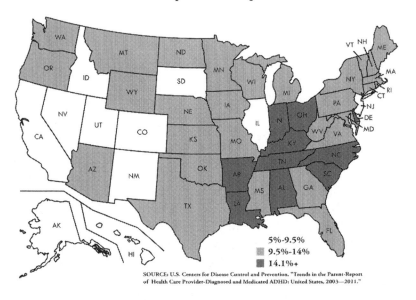

SOURCE: U.S. Centers for Disease Control and Prevention. "Trends in the Parent-Report of Health Care Provider-Diagnosed and Medicated ADHD: United States, 2003—2011."

The Causes of the ADHD Diagnosis Explosion

Why are more children being diagnosed with ADHD? Several factors are influencing this trend to diagnose children with this common behavioral disorder.

Marketing

Pharmaceutical companies have dramatically increased their marketing of ADHD medications to physicians and in some cases consumers. They have also lobbied international governments—for example, Italy and France—to remove restrictions on the sale of stimulants for the treatment of ADHD. Major market forces are dumping significant amounts of money into marketing psychostimulants used to treat ADHD in order to influence doctors' and patients' perceptions of these medications. This savvy and persistent marketing campaign has elevated psychostimulants to the earliest option for ADHD treatment—often at the expense of other proven options. The remarkable increase in ADHD diagnoses and psychostimulant use are both evidence that the two-decade long campaign by pharmaceutical companies to increase ADHD awareness and promote pills as the solution has been extremely effective.

This "disease mongering" has become so rampant that in 2004 and 2005, the British House of Commons expressed concerns that the pharmaceutical industry has encouraged a "pill-for-every-ill" society by categorizing an increasing number of individuals as abnormal and thereby requiring medication.[16] The gift-giving and incentives showered upon physicians by the pharmaceutical industry have drastically influenced physician prescribing patterns, shifting from what is in the patient's best interest to what is in the pharmaceutical companies' best interests.[17,18,19] Although drug marketing is not the only factor in increased ADHD diagnoses, its gratuitous influence cannot be denied.

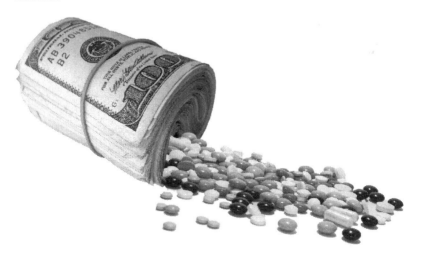

Parents Demand a Diagnosis

Information about ADHD is now readily available at the touch of our fingertips via the Internet. Countless forums, websites, and blogs share what ADHD is and how to determine if you or your child have it. Easy access to information has increased ADHD awareness and provided the ability for parents to identify symptoms in their children. Armed with this information parents go to their physicians, practically guiding him or her to an ADHD diagnosis. Unfortunately, as pointed out in the marketing section above, some of this awareness has increased due to marketing by the pharmaceutical industry that tells parents their child must be medicated to be "normal" again. This myth is perpetuated by financial interests of billion-dollar companies, despite the fact that experts agree that parent behavior therapy should be the first option for children under the age of six with ADHD.[20]

More Distractions for Children

It is estimated that from 1960 to the turn of the century, the use of ADHD medication among children increased a hundred-fold,[21, 22] and some suggest this increase is largely caused by a dramatic increase in "screen" time among children. Captivating screens are found in homes, cars, airplanes, and stores, and they are even carried in the palms of our hands everywhere we go. Increased access to screens has led to overstimulation of children and dysregulation of the normal sleep-wake cycle. In essence, children's brains are so used to being stimulated by technology they require more and more stimulation to be able to focus.

It is believed that the unnaturally stimulating effect of electronic screens and the greater access to these devices may detrimentally affect mental and human health. What exactly are bright LED screens doing? Research suggests that the bright blue-light wavelength emitted by these devices may dysregulate melatonin production, which disrupts normal circadian rhythms and the sleep-wake cycle.[23,24] Irregular sleep-wake cycles result in disrupted sleep, insomnia, and excessive daytime sleepiness.

Additional research has connected a disrupted (or delayed) circadian rhythm to ADHD symptoms.[25,26] In essence, dysregulation of the circadian rhythm leads to poor sleep and an exhausted child, which in turn causes overactivation of the nervous system in the body's efforts to remain alert. Overactivation of the nervous system places body functions out of balance, and that negatively affects memory and attention. This pattern repeats continually and prevents the child from receiving restorative sleep, further compounded by stimulant medications prescribed for the disorder. While this connection has not been established as a definitive cause of ADHD, mounting evidence suggests that more bright screen time leads to attention problems, lack of self-regulation, aggression, and behavioral problems.[27,28,29]

Insurance Policies that Prohibit Proper Diagnosis

Today's pediatricians and family physicians must rapidly diagnose patients and move to the next patient to be profitable. It is typical for primary care physicians to schedule appointments every fifteen minutes, and some hospital physicians are urged to spend only eleven minutes with patients. Indeed, insurance companies, Medicare, and the American Medical Association encourage a short visit of fifteen minutes based on the "relative value units" used by these organizations to calculate doctor's fees. So, instead of spending sufficient time to get adequate information and make a proper diagnosis, doctors are worried about beating the clock to remain profitable.

We have certainly allowed a major disservice to occur to our doctors and the patients they serve by allowing profit-minded organizations to determine what amount of time doctors and patients should spend together. In order to be profitable in these private insurance and Medicare systems, the average physician needs to see about twenty-five patients per day. Accounting for phone calls, e-mails, prescription processing, documenting patient findings, reviewing laboratory results and X-rays, and a dozen or more special consult reports, this doesn't leave more than ten to fifteen minutes per patient to remain profitable. All of these factors lead to too many hurried diagnoses of ADHD entirely based on a hasty visit to the doctor's office instead of a thorough history and proper testing. Increasingly short doctor visits take a toll on patients who receive a quick diagnosis and also increase the likelihood that a drug will be prescribed.[30] It's simply faster—and, therefore, more profitable—to write a prescription and move on to the next patient than to consider other alternative, but viable, treatment options.

Government Policies in Relation to Childhood Education

Stephen Hinshaw, a professor of psychology at the University of California, noticed large discrepancies in ADHD diagnoses across states. For example, over 15 percent of children in North Carolina aged four to seventeen were diagnosed with ADHD in 2007, while in California only 6.2 percent of this same age group was diagnosed. To determine the cause of this discrepancy in the geographic distribution of ADHD, Hinshaw evaluated race, income, diagnostic methods, types of health insurance, cultural ideals, and the geographic areas' perceptions of mental illness. It wasn't until he evaluated educational policies that he found a plausible answer. He discovered that diagnoses with ADHD directly correlated with the introduction of educational policies like the No Child Left Behind Act.[31] As policies were implemented to punish or reward schools for their standardized test scores, ADHD diagnoses increased.

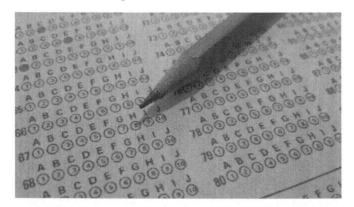

In other words, administrators and teachers were anxious to improve test scores at all costs—even if it meant getting children diagnosed with ADHD so they could be medicated to improve their test performances. Another reason to seek an ADHD diagnosis for a child is the fact that some districts in the United States remove a child's test scores from official school averages if they are diagnosed with ADHD. So poor-performing students may be diagnosed with ADHD simply to avoid their scores counting against the school's average, whether there is a biological disorder or not. Other researchers reported that children residing in states with more stringent school accountability laws are not only more likely to be diagnosed with ADHD, but also they are more likely to be prescribed psychostimulants.[32] In essence, what school administrators are doing is pursuing ADHD diagnoses to remove underperforming children or legally supply them performance-enhancing drugs to improve the school's performance on standardized tests.

DSM versus ICD definition of ADHD

Psychiatrists and physicians in the United States utilize the Diagnostics and Statistical Manual of Mental Disorders (DSM) to classify and diagnose mental disorders. Much of the rest of the world—one hundred countries—relies on the World Health Organization's International Classification of Diseases (ICD) to classify diseases and other health problems. Currently, the DSM definition is more widely accepted, which is slightly broader than the definition contained in the ICD.

ICD-10 definition
- A combination of overactive, poorly modulated behavior with marked inattention and lack of persistent task involvement.
- Symptoms occur prior to six years of age and of long duration.
- Impairment present in two or more settings (e.g. home, classroom, clinic).
- Exclude diagnosis of anxiety disorders, mood-affective disorders, pervasive developmental disorders, and schizophrenia.

DSM-5 definition

- A pattern of behavior, present in multiple settings (e.g. school and home), that can result in social, educational, and occupational performance issues.
- Symptoms occur prior to age twelve and present at least six months.
- Children with at least six symptoms from one of two group criteria: inattentive or hyperactivity and impulsivity. Adolescents and adults with five symptoms present.

  Inattention Symptoms:
  - Often fails to give close attention to details or makes careless mistakes in schoolwork, at work, or with other activities.
  - Often has trouble holding attention on tasks or play activities.
  - Often does not seem to listen when spoken to directly.
  - Often does not follow through on instructions and fails to finish schoolwork, chores, or duties in the workplace (e.g., loses focus, side-tracked).
  - Often has trouble organizing tasks and activities.
  - Often avoids, dislikes, or is reluctant to do tasks that require mental effort over a long period of time (such as schoolwork or homework).
  - Often loses things necessary for tasks and activities (e.g. school materials, pencils, books, tools, wallets, keys, paperwork, eyeglasses, mobile telephones).
  - Is often easily distracted.
  - Is often forgetful in daily activities.

Three types (also called subtypes) of attention deficit disorder (ADD) are currently recognized by the American Psychological Association, and the type diagnosed can change over time as symptoms change:

1. *ADHD, Predominantly inattentive.* More inattention symptoms present, but not hyperactivity-impulsivity, during the last six months.
2. *ADHD, Predominantly hyperactive-impulsive.* More hyperactivity-impulsivity symptoms present, but not inattention, during the last six months.
3. *ADHD, Combined presentation.* Sufficient symptoms of both inattention and hyperactivity-impulsivity present during the last six months.

There are a number of psychological and medical problems that mirror ADHD symptoms, so it is very important that the child be carefully evaluated. It is very possible that a child will meet all the diagnostic criteria for ADHD but have an entirely different problem. Common conditions that could mimic ADHD include depression, anxiety, child abuse or neglect, bipolar disorder, schizophrenia, circadian rhythm disorders, and thyroid dysregulation. It is also possible that one or more of these other conditions may be co-occurring with ADHD. Given these possibilities, the complexity of ADHD, and the variety of disorders that could "look like" ADHD, it is vital that other conditions be ruled out during a comprehensive psychological and medical evaluation.

Conclusion

A variety of factors are influencing the astonishing growth in ADHD diagnoses, and there is not one simple solution to reverse these trends. It will take better parent and teacher/administrator education, reeling in the onslaught of irresponsible marketing by drug companies, more thorough diagnoses from health professionals, and modifications of insurance and government regulations and policies. If action is not taken soon, we will continue to see a rapid increase in children and adults diagnosed with ADHD. Worse, a larger percentage of the population will be medicated with harmful stimulant medications unnecessarily. Take what steps you can now as an individual to stop this slow descent down the slippery slope we are on to an overmedicated society.

2

THE CAUSE OF ADHD—AN ENIGMA SHROUDED IN MYSTERY, YET HIDING IN PLAIN SIGHT

The exact cause of ADHD is not currently known, but it likely stems from several factors, including brain development, genetics, and environmental factors. Many of the neurological mechanisms of ADHD have been known for some time and clinicians are beginning to see a pattern emerge, but like everything that affects human health, ADHD initiates in an individual nature and affects each person differently. This developing pattern is leading us closer to the conclusion that ADHD is predominantly caused by environmental factors (such as exposure to toxins) that triggers neurological and genetic changes and creates the perfect environment for ADHD to occur. This chapter explores a number of the possible causes involved in triggering or exacerbating ADHD symptoms.

It should be noted that just because someone has a gene associated with ADHD does not mean he will absolutely have ADHD. Expression of the genes associated with the condition usually requires something external to "trigger" it—usually diet, activity, or an environmental factor (i.e. toxins). Without this trigger, a person may escape ADHD despite having the genes associated with it. Realistically, myriad factors have been linked to ADHD symptoms, and scientists and medical professionals are still trying to determine which of all these factors are most influential in its development and progression.

Interestingly, autism and ADHD result from very similar mechanisms and differ primarily in the severity of damage to the brain. In many aspects, autism is just a more severe progression of a neurological problem. There is a great deal of overlap between the symptoms of ADHD (i.e. inattention, hyperactivity, impulsivity, sensory processing difficulties, behavior problems, and impaired social skills) and autism spectrum disorder.

However, children with autism are more likely to experience impaired communication skills, struggle to cope with empathy due to feeling other's emotions too intensely, and have greater difficulty engaging with others. Knowing the similarities in the progression of both conditions, it is possible that a person with autism spectrum disorder could benefit from the same interventions that will be outlined in this book. However, his or her response will likely be less obvious and take more time to occur because he or she has more severe neurological impairment in general.

Genetics

Over two thousand studies on ADHD and genetics have been conducted to date, with this number greatly accelerating over the last decade. These studies have produced a compelling amount of evidence that genetics may play a role in ADHD susceptibility. In fact, family and twin studies suggest that ADHD may be inherited up to 80 percent of the time.[33,34] But other research concludes that genetic risks for ADHD play only a minor role and the genetic variants involved are rare.[35] Nevertheless, it is important to review what we currently know about genetics and how they might influence ADHD initiation and severity.

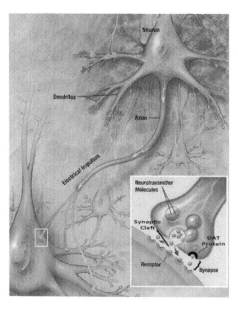

Based on emerging evidence and an improved understand-ing of the human genome, scientists have determined that a number of genes are associated with the development of ADHD.[36] The genes associated with ADHD thus far are involved with the production and balance of dopamine and serotonin, or genes important for psychological and neurological functions.[37,38,39,40,41,42] Variants in these genes cause imbalances in the brain that can trigger ADHD symptoms like inattention, impulsivity, and hyperactivity. Three of the most common genes associated with ADHD in the published literature include DRD4, DRD5, and DAT1 (SLC6A3), although even this association has been mixed in research.[43,44,45,46] Some research finds a strong correlation with variants in these three genes and ADHD, while other research finds these genes are rare in people with ADHD. The inconclusive evidence to implicate one or more specific genes in causing ADHD is largely due to the complexity of ADHD and the myriad factors that influence symptoms.

- o DRD4 (Dopamine Receptor D4) is a protein-coding gene for the D4 subtype of the dopamine receptor involved in dopamine regulation. Dopamine signaling is vital to neurological functions like attention, mood, memory, learning, behavior, and movement. The DRD4 gene is highly variable (called polymorphisms), which can dramatically alter its influence on overall health.
- o DRD5 (Dopamine Receptor D5) also serves to make a protein for the D5 subtype of the dopamine receptor. This cellular receptor is found on brain cells in the limbic system of the brain and has a ten times greater affinity (attraction between two molecules that causes them to combine) than the D1 dopamine subtype.
- o DAT1 (Dopamine Active Transporter 1 Gene), also known as SLC6A3 (Solute Carrier Family 6) creates a protein—dopamine transporter—that is influential in the reuptake of dopamine from the synapse. Dopamine is released into the space between neurons (called the synaptic cleft) and is required for relaying messages between neurons. The protein created by DAT1 regulates the amount of dopamine present in the synaptic cleft and transports it from the synaptic cleft into the neuron for reuse (see image on previous page). DAT1 is a major regulator of dopamine signaling in the brain.

Many of these genetic associations surround copy number variations (CNVs), which are variances in the number of copies of a particular gene from one individual to the next. Until recently, it was generally believed that genes within the human genome were almost always present in pairs (or copies). However, scientists now know that large segments of DNA can have varied numbers of copies. This can be a deletion (only one copy instead of two) or a duplication (three or more copies), and in a few rare instances, the genes can be missing completely. While scientists are still determining the consequences of CNVs, they do know that they play important roles in human disease and drug responses—which also suggests CNVs may influence responses to natural products.[47,48,49,50] Indeed, CNVs may be partly responsible for variations in responses to drug treatments, and why some people experience drastic benefits when using a natural product, while others experience no effect.

COPY NUMBER VARIATION

DELETION
The loss of part of
a chromosome or
sequence of DNA
during DNA replication

DUPLICATION
The duplication of
a sequence of DNA
during DNA replication

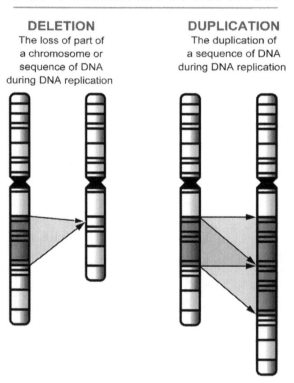

Even if the relationship between genetics and ADHD is proven to be a small causal factor, a better understanding of the genetic association to ADHD could lead to improved diagnosis and treatment options. This is particularly true when you consider the potential role of CNVs in a person's response to dietary supplement and nutritional interventions. An expanded understanding of genetics in relation to ADHD may lead to more effective and individualized management plans and enhance treatment outcomes.

Structural or Functional Brain Changes

The brain consists of three parts: the forebrain (cerebrum, thalamus, and hypothalamus), midbrain (tectum and tegmentum), and hindbrain (cerebellum, pons, and medulla), each of which controls specific functions. The structure of the brain is constantly changing from birth throughout one's lifetime. A number of factors such as physical activity, regular meditation, experiences, music, and amount and duration of stress produce changes to brain structure.[51,52,53,54] In other words, the brain is constantly adapting to experiences, environmental factors, and life itself. Regular structural adaptations produce alterations in the functions and abilities of specific brain regions. Understanding the normal brain structural changes caused by development and aging and those related to disease is important for distinguishing abnormalities that may cause disorders.

Brain imaging techniques have identified disruptions or disturbances in brain circuitry in children with ADHD. The brain consists of billions of neurons, each of which communicates with thousands of other neurons. Brain circuits link neurons together and connect different regions of the brain so they can work together. Every thought, action, and feeling humans experience requires a coordinated effort by many neurons working together. One neuron sends information to another, and that neuron continues the delivery of the message to the next neuron, and so on. This activity allows the brain to process information and then respond appropriately to the information. In children with ADHD, the neural circuits involving concentration, impulse control, motor activity, and inhibitions are often disrupted.

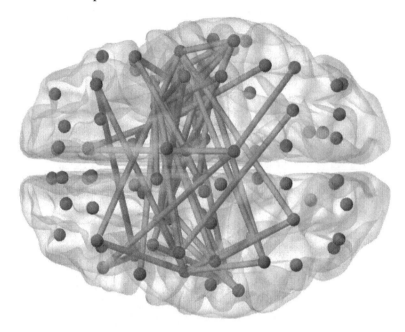

Brain imaging techniques (structural: magnetic resonance imaging and diffusion tensor imaging; functional: magnetic resonance imaging, electroencephalography, and magnetoencephalography) have also identified structural and functional abnormalities in children and adolescents with ADHD, particularly in the prefrontal regions important to attention and motor planning.[55,56,57,58,59,60,61,62] The frontal areas of the brain allow people to suppress inappropriate behavior and thoughts, maintain attention, control movement, preserve memories, and work for reward. Changes in the frontal areas of the brain influence both hemispheres (left and right) of the brain. The right hemisphere of the brain is responsible for regulating attention, impulsivity, and socially responsible behavior. Disruption of this hemisphere due to structural or functional brain changes may lead to hyperactive, disruptive, aggressive, and oppositional behavior.

Scientists have also observed that the brain matures a few years late in youth with ADHD. For example, the cortex of the ADHD brain is developing in a normal pattern, but the development is delayed by about three years. Peak cortex thickness (called cortex maturation) is attained at an average age of 10.5 in children with ADHD, compared to 7.5 years of age among youth without ADHD.[63] Areas at the side of the brain called temporal regions, which play an important role in organizing input from the senses, memory association and formation, speech, and emotional responses, also show delays in development. This would explain why some children grow out of their ADHD symptoms in their teen years and into adulthood—their brain has caught up to their peers, removing obstacles that caused ADHD symptoms.

Another structural abnormality observed in children with ADHD is a reduced volume of gray and white matter in the brain. White matter is whitish nerve tissue within the central nervous system (CNS)—the brain and spinal cord—primarily composed of myelinated nerve fibers called axons. Neurons have wire-like structures—called axons—extending from them that serve to carry signals from the body of the neuron. Myelinated axons are covered with a protective coating called a myelin sheath that gives off a whitish color. This protective coating improves the speed and efficiency with which neurons can conduct signals (kind of like the difference between 10Mbps and 1,000Mbps internet speed). The primary function of white matter is to regulate signals from axons that are used to facilitate communication between neurons.

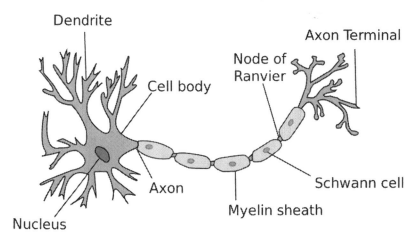

Gray matter is grayish nerve tissue within the central nervous system primarily composed of nerve cell bodies and their dendrites and supportive structures. The cell body of the neuron and tree-like projections (dendrites) are not myelinated and contain capillary blood vessels, which makes them give off a grayish color. Gray matter is found in regions of the CNS that are involved in muscle control, sensory perception (like seeing and hearing), memory, emotions, and speech.

While many children grow out of their ADHD symptoms as they grow older, some continue to have difficulties that persist late into adulthood. Researchers suggest that this may be due to irregularities in gray matter volume as an adult. Young adults with severe ADHD symptoms tend to have less gray matter in the central nervous system, both in localized regions (middle frontal gyrus, cerebellum, and basal ganglia) and widespread areas, but increased gray matter in the temporal and inferior parietal cortices.[64,65,66,67,68] This irregularity in gray matter volume may interfere with the ability to focus attention and increase hyperactivity.

In addition to gray and white matter abnormalities, brain imaging has revealed that people with ADHD have disrupted connectivity in white matter regions of the brain such as the inferior parietal, occipitoparietal, inferior frontal, and inferior temporal complex.[69,70,71] White matter is the connecting link between different brain regions, and thicker or more white matter is associated with a more developed brain. Disruptions in the amount of white matter alter structural connectivity in the brain and therefore cause functional problems like the disruption of neuronal communication. Studies have also identified abnormal myelination of neurons and widespread differences in white matter integrity among adults whose ADHD symptoms persist.[72] Abnormalities in white matter and myelination are associated with greater impulsivity and reduced ability to restrain inappropriate behaviors and emotional responses.

Another disruption in brain communication involves glial cells. Glial cells are the primary immune cells of the central nervous system. They are activated by toxins or pathogens, causing them to migrate to sites of injury or infection in the brain to destroy harmful substances and remove damaged brain cells. They do so largely by releasing chemicals that increase inflammation in the infected/injured area. Glial cells are vital for repair following nerve damage, which makes them important for regeneration of damaged nerves. The brain limits the spread of damage by sealing off the damaged region with glial cells. In addition, glial cells participate in two-way communication with nerve transmitting cells, which suggests they are vital to learning. Proper flow of information among these cells is crucial for forming new connections, strengthening existing connections, and fostering optimal brain function. When glial cells are damaged, disrupted, or overexcited by toxins or pathogens, harmful effects to the brain occur.

Damage to glial cells can occur in the womb or after birth. Moreover, when glial cells are overactivated or activated unnecessarily excess inflammation occurs in the nervous system, which is an underlying cause of a number of neurological disorders. It is when this assault on the brain occurs that genetics may play the most prevalent role in the cause of ADHD. Genetic abnormalities associated with mitochondrial disorders or malfunctions in the body's antioxidant defense system make a child more likely to have severe brain damage. Depending on the person's genetic susceptibility, different areas of the brain may be damaged resulting in different regulation problems and the associated ADHD symptoms. The complexity of the brain and genetic irregularities explain why some ADHD symptoms can be so varied from person to person.

Scientists have also observed that those with ADHD have reduced brain volume in several regions of the brain, including the right anterior frontal region; cerebellum; posterior inferior vermis; splenium of the corpus callosum; total and right cerebral volume; right caudate; right global pallidus; temporal lobe; and pulvinar.[73,74,75,76] A great deal of the irregularities identified appears to affect the right side of the brain. Bearing in mind that the right side of the brain is responsible for regulating attention, impulsivity, and socially responsible behavior, it is easy to see how these abnormalities in brain volume could trigger or exacerbate ADHD symptoms. On average, children with ADHD have 3 to 4 percent smaller brain volume than children without ADHD. Discrepancies in brain volume have been associated with decreased academic achievement.[77] Brain scans demonstrate that the larger the discrepancy in brain volume, the greater the severity of ADHD symptoms in children.

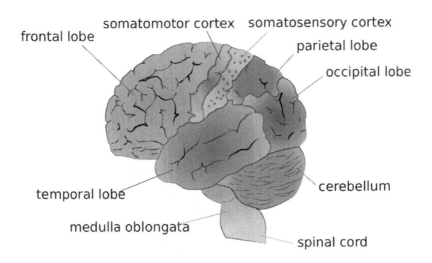

Some evidence suggests that specific regions of the brain may be under- or overactivated, modifying brain electrical activity.[78] Brainwaves are produced by synchronized electrical pulses from masses of neurons communicating with each other. Emotions, behaviors, thoughts, and actions are dependent on this electrical activity and communication. One way to think of brainwaves is to consider them in the context of music. Low-frequency waves (delta waves) are like deeply penetrating bass drum beats, whereas higher frequency (gamma waves) brainwaves are similar to a high-pitched flute. Brainwaves synchronize through harmonics the same way a symphony orchestra—consisting of diverse groups of musical instruments—collaborate to produce beautiful, moving music. Our brainwaves adapt to thoughts, emotions, and physical activity, which alters mood state, energy levels, and state of alertness.

BRAIN WAVES	
Delta waves (less than 4 Hz)	Delta waves are found most often in infants and young children and are associated with the deepest levels of relaxation, meditation, and restorative sleep. They reduce awareness of our external surroundings and are the source of empathy, healing, and regeneration.
Theta waves (4 Hz–7 Hz)	Theta waves occur during deep meditation, profound raw emotions, and light sleep. They act as a gateway to memory and learning. During theta activity, our focus turns inward, producing vivid imagery, intuition, and information held deeply in our subconscious.
Alpha waves (8 Hz–12 Hz)	Alpha waves are present when you are relaxed or idle, and promote a sense of calm. They are dominant during quietly flowing thoughts and aid overall mind/body integration and learning.
Low beta waves (13 Hz–15 Hz)	Low beta waves, or Beta 1, are well-known for their association with a highly attentive, focused concentration.
Mid-range beta waves (15 Hz–18 Hz)	Mid-range beta waves, also known as Beta 2, increase energy, anxious feelings, and performance. They are active during highly complex thought and while integrating new experiences.
High beta waves (18 Hz–40 Hz)	High beta waves, or Beta 3, are linked to high stress levels, excitement, complex thought, anxiety, paranoia, high energy, and intense arousal.
Gamma waves (40 Hz–100 Hz)	Gamma waves are the highest frequency and involved in information processing and cognitive function—memory, learning, and perception. They are present when the mind is quiet and highly active during states of altruism and universal love.

Scientists have observed increased theta and beta brain waves in people with ADHD, or an abnormal theta/beta ratio.[79,80,81] Beta waves are commonly observed while awake and involved in conscious thought and logical thinking. They can be further divided into low, mid, and high beta waves (see graphic). A delicate balance of beta waves is required to focus and complete school or occupational tasks. Theta brain waves are often present when engaged in complex problem solving and the presence of theta waves during normal awake states—commonly present in individuals with ADHD—may suggest problems with focus and attention.

BRAIN ACTIVATION PATTERNS IN ADULTS AND CHILDREN/ADOLESCENTS WITH ADHD[7]		
Age	**Overactive regions**	**Underactive regions**
Children & adolescents	▪ right angular gyrus ▪ middle occipital gyrus ▪ posterior cingulate cortex ▪ midcingulate cortex	▪ right parietal region ▪ right temporal region ▪ frontal regions (bilaterally) ▪ putamen (bilaterally)
Adults	▪ right angular gyrus ▪ middle occipital gyrus	▪ middle frontal gyrus ▪ right central sulcus ▪ precentral gyrus

EEG (electroencephalogram) tests provide an objective way to help distinguish the various subtypes of ADHD—inattentive and combination subtypes—by measuring alpha and beta brain waves. Scientists have found that those with inattentive ADHD have the least ability to suppress alpha waves—something necessary to filter out visual "noise" and use cues to make a decision.[82] Those with combination subtypes of ADHD suppressed beta waves the least, which could cause difficulty in using cues to prepare a motor response (voluntary movement in response to stimuli) during a task. Brainwave balance must be maintained to realize optimum emotional and mental health. Overarousal of specific brain areas can lead to anxiety, sleep disorders, chronic nerve pain, impulsivity, and nightmares. Underarousal of specific brain areas can result in inattention, insomnia, and chronic pain disorders. Interestingly, ADHD brains demonstrate both under- and overarousal. One effective way to retrain and balance brainwave patterns is through meditation (refraining from concentration and intentional thinking), which increases theta and alpha activity.[83,84] Increased theta and alpha brainwaves make optimum mental health more likely. People with ADHD—but really all people—should set aside daily time to meditate quietly to improve brainwave balance and, therefore, brain activity and function.

Brain injury

Preliminary evidence suggests that there may be a relationship between ADHD and traumatic brain injuries (TBI) that occurred during childhood.[85,86,87] However, symptoms of ADHD and TBI are so similar they are often hard to distinguish. Traditionalists argue that ADHD is a developmental disorder and can't be caused by a TBI, and that in reality TBI is simply more common in children with ADHD because of their decreased motor skills. But other experts contend that an acquired form of ADHD— often referred to as secondary attention deficit hyperactivity disorder, or SADHD—may occur following a TBI because of dramatic alterations in psychoneurological function.[88] This debate is similar to whether the chicken came before the egg or vice versa, and we may never have a definitive conclusion.

Evidence has been mixed to support either side of the argument. Children diagnosed with ADHD before experiencing a TBI are more likely to experience severe and persistent ADHD symptoms than children who experience a TBI that do not have ADHD.[89,90] In other words, if a child has ADHD and then suffers a TBI, he or she may experience more severe and long-lasting symptoms. On the contrary, scientists only observed a modest increase in ADHD-like symptoms post-injury (TBI)—14.5% at twelve months and 18.3% at twenty-four months in children without an ADHD diagnosis before the injury occurred. Other research supports a link between suffering a TBI and ADHD, including studies that show that TBI causes alterations in white matter connectivity and axon damage.[91] These brain alterations could certainly lead to disrupted or less-than-optimal brain communication and signaling, so it may contribute to a diagnosis of ADHD. Whether brain injuries cause SADHD or ADHD makes children more prone to TBI will continue to be a topic of debate until more research is completed that considerably supports one side or another.

Chemical Imbalances in the Brain

Another possible causal factor of ADHD is chemical imbalances in the brain, although recently the scientific community has instead pointed to structural and functional brain changes as the more likely culprit. For years, it was believed that delayed development of certain dopaminergic (involving, related to, or activated by dopamine) neural pathways and imbalances of key neurochemicals—dopamine, noradrenaline, and glutamate— were the most likely cause of ADHD.[92,93,94,95,96,97,98] Drugs used for ADHD target these imbalances in neurochemicals. Genetic variations (polymorphisms) may also influence these imbalances of essential neural chemicals. Polymorphisms in specific genes may cause dopamine to be reabsorbed (reuptaking) from synapses too quickly and before it can do its job. Similar patterns may occur with norepinephrine (also called noradrenaline), leading to insufficient norepinephrine levels in the brain. A lack of key neurotransmitters leaves people with ADHD feeling understimulated, unrewarded, and often inattentive.

Early studies that suggested that disruption of dopamine and noradrenaline balance can interrupt the dopamine reward pathway and trigger impulsivity and inattention convinced researchers that it was the underlying cause of ADHD.[99,100] Glutamate is another neurotransmitter that may be involved in ADHD and considered to be the most important neurotransmitter for brain function. Virtually all excitatory (stimulating to the brain) neurons in the central nervous system interact with glutamate, and more than half of brain synapses release glutamate. Scientists have identified polymorphisms in genes related to glutamate, such as GRM1, GRM5, GRM7, and

GRM8, which substantiates the involvement of glutamate as an important pathway in ADHD.[101,102]

A complex interaction between dopamine, noradrenaline, and glutamate exists in the brain, which regulates overall neurotransmitter activity. Increased glutamate levels and glutamate signaling influences how quickly our behavior subsequently changes to external events. Excessive signaling promotes unnecessary responsiveness that can cause a constant shift in attention. Think of the dog Dug from Pixar's movie *Up*, and how his attention shifted at a whim. However, as more research surfaces that suggests that structural and functional alterations in the key areas of the brain—areas involved in proper neuronal function and the routing and processing of sensory stimuli—are more likely the leading cause of ADHD symptoms, the chemical-imbalance theory is beginning to lose support. Instead, other factors like brain abnormalities and environmental factors lead to the neurochemical imbalances.

Toxins—Lead, Food Additives, and Food Dyes

Few mainstream medical professionals are willing to admit that toxins play a causal role in ADHD, but science is emerging to suggest that toxins may be a contributing factor in symptom severity and, at the very least, affect brain development and function.[103,104] Indeed, the experience of some clinicians suggests that toxins may be the primary trigger and far outweight any genetic risks. Toxins that have the ability to disrupt delicate balances in the neuroendocrine system are of particular concern. The nervous and endocrine systems often act together to regulate a number of physiological processes in the human body. The hypothalamus is the link between the two systems and stimulates the pituitary gland to release hormones. The endocrine system is so tightly controlled that it relies on hormone concentrations of a trillionth of a gram to maintain balance in the womb. With such a narrow band to work within, it is easy to see how exposure to even small doses of endocrine-disrupting toxins can alter genetic expression, interfere with hormone function, and cause subtle to serious disruption in fetal brain development.[105,106,107,108,109]

COMMON ENDOCRINE-DISRUPTING CHEMICALS

Toxin	Commonly found in
BPA	Plastics marked as PC or recycle #7, epoxy resins, eyeglasses, lining of metal
Dioxin	Animal foods, air, water, bleached coffee filters, products with triclosan, chlorine bleach, cigarette smoke
Atrazine	Herbicides, insecticides, water, air
Phthalates	Personal care products, perfume, nail polish, pharmaceuticals, plastic wrap, food packaging, cleaning products
Perchlorates	Air, soil, vegetables, fruits, legumes, milk, alcoholic beverages, infant foods, spices, water, pool chemicals, chewing tobacco, cleaning products
PBDEs	Flame-resistant items, furniture, carpet, upholstery, vehicles, household dust
PFCs	Nonstick cookware, stain-resistant carpet and fabrics, food packaging (popcorn bags, fast-food wrappers), soil, water
Pesticides	Nonorganic produce
Glycol Ethers	Household cleaning products, cosmetics, pharmaceuticals, sunscreen, dyes, paints, cleaners, adhesives
Fluoride	Drinking water, toothpaste, oral care products
Toluene	Paint, paint thinners, nail polish, synthetic fragrances, adhesives, vehicle emissions
Lead	Food, water, air, cosmetics, hair dyes, paint (prior to 1978), plumbing, ceramics, batteries
Arsenic	Food, air, water
Methylmercury	Food, air, water, dental amalgams, vaccines

Fetuses' and newborns's abilities to metabolize, detoxify, and eliminate many toxins is different from that of adults, which makes them more sensitive to their toxic effects. Immature organs—like the liver and kidneys—cannot remove toxins as well as an adult's mature organs. Rapidly developing organ systems—like the lungs and central nervous system—are especially vulnerable to toxic insults. If too many toxins are present as these vital systems develop, it can result in widespread damaging effects.

Physical size is also a factor, creating a greater exposure to toxins per pound of body weight. It takes less exposure to a toxin to produce adverse effects in children than adults because of their size difference. In other words, adults may not experience adverse effects from a specific amount of toxins, but a child will at the same exposure level.

In addition, infants have a higher respiratory rate (more breaths per minute) than adults, which may increase inhalation exposure of toxins and the amounts that enter the respiratory and general circulation. Active older children also engage in more physical activity than adults, which leads to a higher breathing rate and greater respiratory system exposure to toxins. Once inside the respiratory system, toxins may migrate to the bloodstream and into general circulation. All of these factors lead to unique vulnerabilities to toxins among children that play significant roles in children's health.

One of the most critical times that toxins can interfere with brain development is throughout the first trimester of pregnancy. During this time, the developing baby is undergoing a complex process—directed by genes, hormones, and neuroendocrine chemicals—that organizes cellular structures and functional features, and establishes connections (called synapses) between neurons. The release of precise amounts of thyroid hormones at defined times plays a critical role in the development of the brain. Thyroid hormones trigger genes that direct myelination and provide timing signals for maturation of brain structures at specific stages of development. The fetus has two potential sources of thyroid hormone—its own thyroid (beginning around week twelve) and its mother's thyroid. Inadequate or disrupted thyroid hormone levels in the womb may cause delayed brain maturation and irregularities in brain white matter. It is vital that the proper amounts of thyroid hormone be transported across the placenta for the brain to develop correctly.[110,111,112,113]

During the first few years of life, a child's brain is still developing and forming an astonishing seven hundred new neural connections every second.[114] Connections are formed through the experiences and thoughts of the child. Experiences require thought, which utilizes brain cells and forms new connections. The more a child uses a connection, the stronger it becomes, leading to the improved ability to perform a task or specific function. A great example is learning to ride a bike. At first the child is wobbly and has great difficulty propelling the bike forward without falling over. Stronger connections in the brain are formed the more the child practices. Eventually he or she has little trouble riding a bike because the brain has adapted to the child's experiences.

Similarly, connections can be weakened and break down (even disappear) when they are not used. If a child learns to play the piano and then quits for a few years, the brain connections to piano playing become weaker due to lack of use. The good news is these connections can be reestablished and strengthened if the child dedicates time to piano practice again. The greater the length of the break from the piano, the more time that will be required to strengthen these connections. It is imperative that exposures to toxins be minimized as key connections are being formed throughout childhood.

Exposure to toxins during this critical time of connection development may be responsible for widespread behavioral and cognitive problems. This is because toxins can disrupt and scramble normal patterns of neuronal connections in the brain. In fact, some toxins trigger a cascade of events that leads to an overabundance of dendrites.[115] Dendrite growth and development is a delicate process and the presence of toxins disrupts proper development, leading to impaired connections. Some toxins of which exposure is linked to ADHD and exacerbation of symptoms include lead, sodium benzoate, organophosphates (bug sprays and pesticides), BPA (bisphenol A), nitrate-based food preservatives, red food dyes, manganese, fluoride, chlorpyrifos and DDT (pesticides), tetrachloroethylene (a solvent), and the polybrominated diphenyl ethers (flame retardants).

Lead

Of the toxins associated with ADHD, lead appears to have the strongest correlation with diagnosis of the disorder.[116,117,118,119] Studies suggest that lead may reduce both attention and the ability to inhibit inappropriate behavioral responses. Higher blood concentrations of lead have been associated with triggering ADHD-specific symptoms in children not previously diagnosed with ADHD.[120] Interestingly the study authors found that lead was more strongly associated with triggering ADHD symptoms than it was with decreasing IQ. Another study found that even low blood levels of lead increased the risk of ADHD symptoms in children.[121] Lead blood levels over 2.17μg/dL have a greater risk of developing ADHD when compared to children with lower lead blood levels.[122] The amount of evidence linking lead to ADHD symptoms can't be ignored.

Research findings that childhood exposure to lead causes structural alterations in the brain add credence to the claim that toxins may play a causal role in ADHD. Scientists have observed that adverse cognitive and behavioral outcomes correlate with reductions in brain gray matter in the prefrontal cortex and anterior cingulate cortex caused by childhood exposure to lead.[123] Further substantiating this correlation is the fact that childhood exposure to lead is associated with decreased white matter connectivity and altered myelination.[124,125] Both of these structural and functional changes to the brain caused by lead have been linked to ADHD symptoms. Since structural and functional alterations of the brain are currently considered by many experts to be the most likely cause of ADHD, the picture becomes much clearer that toxicity is able to influence ADHD risk and development.

Polychlorinated Biphenyls

Polychlorinated biphenyls (PCBs) are chemicals widely used in the past in a number of products, such as lubricants, insulation, electrical equipment, and coatings. Growing concerns over the safety of PCBs lead to their ban in many countries during the 1970s. However, many regions of the world are still contaminated with these chemicals, and their legacy of harm continues far past their ban in the 1970s. A number of studies have associated exposure to PCBs in the womb to behavioral problems and hyperactivity—two key ADHD symptoms—in children.[126,127,128,129] Children with ADHD who are exposed to PCBs are at increased risk of impaired attention and memory, but especially impaired ability to inhibit inappropriate responses to situations.[130] Even adults exposed to indoor air contaminated with PCBs show decreased attention and an altered emotional state.[131] These attention deficits associated with PCBs may be due to adverse effects on thyroid function and brain development.[132,133,134] By altering thyroid and brain function, PCBs contribute to ADHD symptoms and possibly to its cause.

Food Preservatives and Food Dyes

Another consideration that could possibly aggravate or trigger ADHD symptoms is the preservative sodium benzoate and food dyes. Sodium benzoate is a man-made chemical produced by combining benzoic acid (naturally found in some fruits and spices) with sodium hydroxide (a highly reactive inorganic base chemical). It is found in thousands of products like soda, fruit juice, vinegar, wine, pickles, and salad dressings. This harmful preservative is linked to DNA damage and may combine with vitamin C to form a carcinogenic agent called benzene, which may increase the risk of leukemia and aplastic anemia.[135,136,137,138]

Food dyes (artificial colors) create a more appealing color for products made for consumption—such as yellow no. 6, yellow no. 5, red no. 3, red no. 40, blue no. 1, and green no. 3. Researchers in the United Kingdom found that artificial colors and/or sodium benzoate obtained from diet increased the risk of hyperactivity in three-year-old and eight- to nine-year-old children.[139] However, other studies have only associated increased ADHD symptoms in specific subsets of children with a genetic polymorphism (natural variations in a gene, DNA sequence, or chromosome) that involves histamine degradation, or in other words, more susceptible children.[140,141] While focusing on food dyes or preservatives as a single cause of ADHD is foolish, the research does merit removal of or limiting both dyes and preservatives in the diet of children with ADHD, and even among those without a current diagnosis.

Pesticides

Organophosphates (like chlorpyrifos) and pyrethroid compounds are the most widely used pesticide chemicals in the world. Organophosphates work by disrupting the enzyme acetylcholinesterase, which is vital for regulating nerve signals. Damage to the nervous system leads to the death of the pest. Pyrethroids (the chemical used for the majority of household insecticides) are considered less toxic than organophosphates but still work by disrupting nervous system function. Most research suggests that exposure to organophosphates after birth is more likely to cause behavioral problems and poor motor skills in children than prenatal exposure. A study of 1,139 children found that children with higher urinary levels of the organophosphate dialkyl phosphate (DAP) were more likely to have the hyperactive/impulsive subtype of ADHD.[142] The risk of ADHD was doubled among children with organophosphate levels higher than the median average. Other scientists report that prenatal exposure to organophosphate pesticides leads to mental developmental delays, attentional problems, ADHD, and developmental problems in children at age three.[143] An additional study also found a two-fold increased risk of ADHD in children with higher levels of the pesticide pyrethroid.[144] At the very least, these studies should raise awareness of the risks to children associated with pesticides and encourage parents to consider organic options for produce and other food products.

A different type of pesticide that is also of concern is DDT (dichlorodiphenyltrichloroethane), which is an organochloride pesticide. It was first developed in the 1940s, but by the 1950s, regulatory actions were being enacted to prohibit its use because of mounting evidence that it was harmful to animals and humans. However, the World Health Organization still recommends its use today as an indoor pesticide to control the spread of malaria transmitted by disease-carrying mosquitoes. Evidence connects organochlorine pesticide exposure, both prenatal and postnatal, to adverse neurological affects in children, including ADHD symptoms (decreased alertness and inattention).[145,146,147] The more we learn about chemicals exposures prenatally and during childhood, the more we discover that the chemical world we live in is taking a negative toll on the health of children and adults. While it is impossible to eliminate exposure to chemicals, one can certainly take steps to reduce exposures by choosing organic produce and foods, filter drinking and shower water, using natural fabrics (cotton, silk, wool, hemp, etc.), include more houseplants in your home, and use green products (household cleaners, personal care products, paints, etc.).

Bisphenol A (BPA)

BPA (bisphenol A) is a synthetic chemical found in polycarbonate plastics and resins that has been used since the 1960s. Evidence suggests that BPA disrupts the production of endocrine hormones and may impair brain development.[148] Disruption of this system can cause dramatic changes in myriad body functions because the endocrine system releases hormones involved in growth and development, internal balance of body systems, blood sugar and mineral balance, metabolism, reproduction, responses to stimuli, and much, much more. Many manufacturers substitute a closely related chemical, BPS (bisphenol S), for BPA, but concerns that this compound may be equally harmful are increasing.[149,150] Both prenatal and childhood exposure to BPA has been linked to aggressive and hyperactive behavior in boys.[151,152] Scientists theorize that BPA affects boys more than girls because of its effects on male hormone levels and its estrogenic effects. While the research is currently far from definitive enough to say BPA and BPS cause ADHD, it would be wise for pregnant women and children to limit their exposure to these harmful chemicals associated with behavioral problems and altered brain development.

Phthalates

Phthalates—a group of chemicals that improve the flexibility and durability of plastics—are another group of chemicals that may play a role in ADHD symptoms. Studies have found that higher phthalate concentrations in the urine of children are associated with increased ADHD symptoms and an increased risk of ADHD.[153,154] The risk appears to be greatest if the exposure occurs prenatally, which suggests that something as simple as applying nail polish—high in phthalates—during pregnancy could increase ADHD risk in the mother's offspring. Again, the sensible thing to do is to limit phthalate exposure as much as possible.

Fluoride

Fluoride has been passed off as the tooth-saving miracle for decades, despite the mounting evidence that it may cause more harm than good. Many communities—about two-thirds of the US population—are forced to drink fluoridated tap water despite objections to this compulsory practice. Now, research has strongly associated fluoridated water to a higher prevalence of ADHD.[155] Remarkably scientists estimate that 131,000 new cases of ADHD occurred in 2011 for every 1 percent increase in the portion of the population drinking fluoridated water. This adds to existing research that concluded fluoridated water may adversely affect learning, memory, and IQ.[156,157] If you live in an area that provides fluoridated water, you may want to think twice about drinking it.

Manganese

The connection of the heavy metal lead to ADHD was discussed earlier, and research suggests that it is not the only metal that may be connected to hyperactivity. Manganese is a gray-white metal and element found widely in the earth's crust, soil, and water. It is also a key mineral for brain and nervous system function, and helps form connective tissues, bones, and sex hormones. However, abnormal concentrations of manganese in the brain, particularly the basal ganglia, is linked to neurological disorders. While not as conclusive as the lead connection, the manganese-ADHD connection is worth mentioning. Scientists have observed that an unhealthy buildup of manganese may diminish intellectual function, impair motor skills, reduce attention, and cause hyperactivity.[158,159,160] This research is very preliminary and should be viewed cautiously until further research suggests a more definite link to ADHD.

Basal Ganglia and Related Structures of the Brain

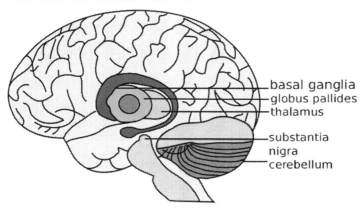

There is no end to the number of chemicals a child could possibly be exposed to these days, and avoiding all of these chemicals is just not feasible. However, a concerted effort to be aware of these chemicals linked to behavioral disorders and ADHD and to reduce exposure to them as much as possible is vital for children's health.

Birth Complications

Some studies suggest that a difficult pregnancy or complications during birth may increase the risk of ADHD. Sometimes an external factor may not be the cause of a condition, but it could increase the risk of it. This may be the case with pregnancy complications being associated with increased risk of ADHD in offspring. For example, research suggests that high blood pressure during pregnancy, bleeding before the birth of the baby, post-term deliveries, extended delivery times, and anything that may reduce the baby's oxygen supply during birth may increase the risk of ADHD.[161,162,163] Even excess maternal stress and anxiety or being induced versus naturally going into labor have been linked to increased risk of ADHD in children.[164,165,166] These factors may damage the brain or alter its function. Pregnancy and birth complications certainly don't guarantee that your child will have ADHD, but they are factors to be conscious of. At the very least, it highlights the need to offer psychological and social support to mothers who experience stress during pregnancy.

Extreme Neglect, Abuse, or Social Deprivation

Research over the last decade has linked child abuse, neglect, and social deprivation to ADHD. It is clear that family environments play an important role in the development of and degree of ADHD symptoms. Many children who are diagnosed with ADHD live in households and neighborhoods where violence and relentless stress is commonplace. Parents of these children find them difficult to manage, and teachers describe them as disruptive, impulsive, hyperactive, misbehaved, and inattentive. These types of environments seem to be a perfect storm for generating children with ADHD symptoms. Whether these family dynamics and factors are causal, play an exacerbating role, or simply provide evidence that children with ADHD are more likely to be abused is yet to be fully determined.

What is clear is that children who are abused are more likely to be aggressive, hostile, angry, impulsive, and externalize their behaviors (negative behaviors directed toward other people or things);[167,168,169] and parents of children with ADHD experience more stress and have more dysfunctional relationships with their children.[170,171,172,173] In addition, children with ADHD are at a significantly greater risk of experiencing poverty, divorce, violence, and family substance abuse.[174] Interestingly, abused children tend to get diagnosed with ADHD earlier than non-abused children.[175] Either way, this data suggests that greater emphasis should be placed on parent education when ADHD is diagnosed.

Some research suggests that children who experience traumatic events or abuse have a higher rate of occupational defiance disorder co-occurring with ADHD, or ADHD alone.[176,177] But this may come down to the chicken and egg debate—whether ADHD triggered the abuse/traumatic event or the abuse/traumatic event caused the ADHD. Indeed, scientists have reported that 60 percent of children with ADHD included in a cross-sectional study had experienced neglect and 35 percent experienced psychological abuse.[178] Adults with ADHD are also more likely to report that they were physically or sexually abused as a child.[179] Women with ADHD are almost 2.5 times more likely to report they were sexually abused when compared to women without ADHD; while men with ADHD were almost twice as likely to report sexual abuse.[180] Similar findings for physical abuse were reported, with women diagnosed with ADHD more than twice as likely to report abuse, and men with ADHD about 33 percent more likely to report abuse. This is a significant amount of abuse that needs to be considered and addressed through appropriate counseling and behavioral therapy.

Adding to the complexity of link between ADHD and abuse is the fact that, in some cases, victims of child abuse or neglect may display ADHD symptoms that are difficult to distinguish from actual ADHD. It is easy to understand how physical abuse could potentially trigger ADHD because of the potential for brain damage, but the damaging effects of psychological abuse and neglect cannot be overlooked. Indeed, psychological abuse may lead to enduring negative effects that harm brain development, which in turn causes undesirable behaviors.[181,182] We know that our brains are sculpted by our early experiences, so abuse must be acknowledged as a possible causal factor in ADHD.

Prenatal Environmental Tobacco Smoke (ETS) Exposure

Environmental tobacco smoke (ETS) is a huge problem for those who choose not to smoke. It is now abundantly clear that smoking is destructive to human health, but some are unwillingly exposed to smoking through inhalation of ETS (a mixture of chemicals exhaled by smokers or released by burning tobacco products). A number of studies have linked ADHD symptoms to exposure to ETS before birth, even when other factors such as exposure to birth and a family history of ADHD are controlled for.[183,184,185,186,187,188,189] Tighter regulations and restrictions on smoking may be necessary to reduce compulsory exposure to harmful chemicals emitted by cigarettes, cigars, pipes, and even electronic cigarettes.

ETS interferes with cellular communication, alters brain structure and function, impairs brain development, and negatively influences genes that have the potential to affect multiple generations.[190,191,192] Scientists have observed that prenatal ETS exposure significantly increases the risk of ADHD, and this risk increases even more when children are exposed to more than one neurotoxin during childhood.[193,194] E-cigarettes are not free of harmful effects, despite claims from the manufacturers. Ultrafine particles are released during vaping that can be deposited in the lungs of both the smoker and those who inhale the ETS, which can increase lung inflammation.[195] The obvious conclusion here is to quit smoking if you are pregnant and avoid ETS while pregnant as much as possible to reduce the risk of ETS-triggered ADHD. In addition, smokers should avoid smoking (or vaping) in places where children— particularly developing children—are present.

Vaccines

While discredited scientists with falsified data have been a problem in attempts to link vaccinations to ADHD and autism, surveys do suggest a strong correlation with vaccinations and neurological disorders. Generation Rescue commissioned a survey to determine whether vaccines increase the risk of neurological disorders, like ADHD and autism, in children.

More than 17,600 children were included in the survey, of which 991 were described as completely unvaccinated. The research survey concluded that vaccinated boys were 155 percent more likely to have a neurological disorder, 224 percent more likely to have ADHD, and 61 percent more likely to have autism, when compared to their unvaccinated peers.[196] Interestingly, the same correlation was not observed in girls, with vaccinated and unvaccinated girls having similar prevalence of neurological disorders, ADHD, and autism. Although a survey is far from definitive proof that vaccines cause ADHD, the significant increase of its occurrence in vaccinated boys can't be ignored; nor can the reports and observations of open-minded clinicians.

Some of the concern surrounding vaccinations and their potential to harm the neurological system involves their destructive additives and preservatives. Scientists are now beginning to link neurological disorders to toxins in vaccines like ethanol and light to heavy metals (aluminum and ethyl mercury).[197] This is not surprising considering these are all neurotoxins that have been shown to cause nervous system damage at sufficient doses.[198,199,200] Medical professionals and scientists may debate the degree of toxicity among the different forms of these neurotoxins or the levels at which they are harmful, but the fact is they can all cause harm and evidence suggests some people are more susceptible to this damage (fetuses and individuals with certain genes).

Excess ethanol (2-Phenoxyethanol) exposure can lead to serious damage of the entire nervous system, but particularly the brain. Imaging techniques demonstrate that excess ethanol can cause brain shrinkage, interfere with neurotransmitter signaling and function, and damage neural cells. A certain level of exposure (acute or chronic) must occur for damage to happen. However, as immunization schedules rapidly grow in scope and number, neurological damage caused by exposure to vaccine additives and preservatives becomes a greater concern and risk.

Mercury is particularly harmful because it penetrates and damages the blood-brain barrier rapidly, which disrupts its function to keep harmful substances out of the brain. In addition, it disrupts mitochondrial function and dysregulates the structure, communication, and function of neurons. Symptoms of neurological damage caused by mercury include headache, cognitive and motor dysfunction, tremors, insomnia, memory loss, and neuromuscular effects. Scientists observed significantly increased risk of neurological disorders—including ADHD—from the cumulative effect of the thimerosal-containing hepatitis B vaccine (T-HBV), which exposes infants to 12.5 to 25 mcg of organic mercury per dose (for a total of up to 75 mcg over the course of the three required doses).[201] Understanding the risks that mercury poses to children, thimerosal was eliminated from childhood vaccines in the United States in 2001. However, multi-dose vaccines (like the flu shot) still contain thimerosal as a preservative. No sane person would continually subject their body to the toxic effects of mercury on a regular basis. It really has no place in the human body or in vaccines.

While the use of thimerosal has been eliminated in single dose vaccines, the use of aluminum as a preservative has increased. Aluminum is added to vaccines to increase the host's response to the antigen (causes the body to create antibodies in response to the virus being injected more quickly). A number of vaccines contain aluminum (hepatitis A, hepatitis B, DTaP, Hib, pneumococcal, and HPV vaccines). Aluminum is added to vaccines to reduce production cost, supposedly because less of the antigen is required to produce an immune response. The FDA states that people with impaired kidney function, or premature infants, who are exposed to aluminum levels greater than 4 to 5 mcg/kg per day are at a greater risk of central nervous system toxicity, and tissue loading may occur at even lower rates of administration.[202] To put this in perspective a two month old baby is about eleven pounds, giving us a daily maximum of 25 mcg of aluminum (using the above figures of 4 to 5 mcg/kg/day). The current immunization schedule for a two month old calls for hepatitis B, RV (rotavirus), DTaP (diphtheria, tetanus, and pertussis), Hib (*Haemophilus influenzae* type b), PCV (pneumococcal), and IPV (polio) vaccines, which can easily expose a two month old to more than 1,000 mcg of aluminum depending on the brand and combinations used. One must ask, why are vaccines exempt from this maximum limit?

Some experts believe that the risks of adverse reactions to vaccines or vaccine damage may increase if a child receives a vaccination when an active illness is present or when medications (like acetaminophen) are used at the same time. According to one study, parents were four times more likely to report adverse reactions to vaccines in their children when they gave them acetaminophen to manage the fever.[203] Adverse reactions or vaccine damage may be the result of the toxins within vaccines disrupting the body's ability to create antioxidants and neutralize free radicals. Without the ability to handle the onslaught of toxins and free radicals a state of oxidative stress occurs, resulting in damage to the cell membrane, mitochondria, and DNA. Consequently, abnormal expression of genes in relation to development and neuronal communication, and an increase in neuron cell death may occur. However, current research suggests that this cascade of events and complex interaction with acetaminophen, vaccines, and active illnesses is most likely to affect children who are more genetically susceptible.[204] If you choose to vaccinate your children, it would be wise to avoid giving them acetaminophen within several days of the vaccine and to avoid vaccination when an active illness is present.

These days' vaccines seem as mandatory as taxes and death, so there is huge profits for vaccine manufacturers. Infants and children line up at doctor's offices to be injected with multiple vaccines on an expected schedule. Those who don't are ridiculed as anti-science extremists who put world populations at risk for the next health epidemic. Manufacturers are often found to be behind the spread of misinformation and poor science so that they can protect windfall profits. All of this leads to very muddy waters that make it difficult to see clearly so parents can make an educated and informed decision. Hopefully the controversy will be put to bed with valid and honest science, not funded or pushed by vaccine manufacturers, in the near future. Until then, we are left wondering to what expense our children are being subjected to the additives and preservatives contained in vaccines.

Conclusion

When you consider all the possible causes and triggers of ADHD symptoms, it can be a bit overwhelming. Some of the theories are controversial, and some experts even suggest that ADHD may be at least a consequence of our fast-paced, overly stressed lives. Ongoing research will continue to reveal new links to ADHD, and may someday reveal the most common causes of this widespread behavioral disorder. In reality, a single cause is not likely; rather, scientists may discover a set of causes that affect brain function, development, and genetic expression. Until then, it is important to consider multiple factors as a risk for, or cause or trigger of ADHD and do what is within your power to mitigate these factors.

3

THE WESTERN APPROACH TO ADHD TREATMENT

Parents may be overwhelmed when their child receives an ADHD diagnosis. They likely have multiple questions and concerns regarding what is the best option to help their child. There is no cure for ADHD, and it is considered a chronic condition that will require long-term management. Finding the right option is crucial to managing ADHD and to your child's future success. Parents should work closely with everyone involved in the child's life—family members, teachers, therapists, health professionals, ecclesiastical leaders, neighbors, and coaches—to improve the likelihood of successful management and help others understand the child's needs. The ultimate goal of treatment is to improve your child's ability to pay attention, reduce hyperactivity, maintain meaningful relationships with peers and adults, and control impulsive behavior.

Western medicine largely relies on three primary treatment options for ADHD: behavior therapy, medications, and school accommodations and interventions. Frequently combinations of the three are employed, but this largely depends on the child's age and severity of symptoms. The American Academy of Pediatrics (AAP) recommends behavioral therapy as the first treatment option for preschool-aged children (four to five years of age) before the administration of medication. This includes therapy for the parent and possibly the teacher. A combination of behavior therapy and medication is the preferred treatment for elementary-aged children (six to eleven years old). Medication or behavior therapy can also be used alone in elementary-aged children. The AAP recommends medication as the first line of treatment for adolescents (twelve to eighteen years of age), preferably combined with behavioral therapy. The suggested course of action will be determined by your child's health professional.

Behavior Therapy

Behavior therapy, also called behavioral modification, is a common type of mental health counseling (psychotherapy) that replaces negative habits with positive ones. Its primary focus is the alteration of the external environment and the physiological function of the internal environment to cause behavior change. It addresses specific problem behaviors by increasing positive attention, establishing routines at home, and structuring time. Cognitive behavior therapy is a similar therapy and offshoot of behavior therapy. By contrast, cognitive therapy focuses on thinking as the factor that will create change. It helps children with ADHD recognize inaccurate thinking patterns so that they can more effectively assess challenging situations and respond to them in a more positive manner. It is particularly helpful to improve social skills and for parent training. Because these two forms of psychological therapy are more similar than dissimilar they will not be differentiated for the purpose of this text; rather the term behavior therapy will be used.

Behavior therapy is based on the theories of classical and operant conditioning. Classical conditioning suggests that all behavior is learned, and faulty learning (conditioning) causes abnormal behavior. To correct the abnormal or negative behavior, an individual must be taught the correct or acceptable behavior. In other words, a response to a situation is learned and repeated through association, and behavior therapy aims to disconnect the situational association with the negative learned response. Operant conditioning utilizes reinforcement, punishment, shaping (the gradual training of a person to respond a specific way to situations by reinforcing the desired response), and modeling (learning by imitating what has been observed) techniques to alter behavior. In the end, the goal is to teach and reinforce positive behaviors and eliminate negative learned behaviors and responses.

BEHAVIOR THERAPY TECHNIQUES APPROVED BY THE AAP

Positive Reinforcement
This technique works well for young children who require immediate gratification for positive behaviors. Small rewards—treats, stickers, TV time, etc.—are provided to the child in exchange for compliance with requests.

Reward System
This technique is more suited for older children who understand long-term goals and rewards. As part of this system, a chart with goals is placed in a visible location. When the child completes a goal, a mark is placed next to the goal, and when all goals are achieved, a bigger reward is offered.

Time-out
Time-outs are best reserved for a cooling-off period rather than a punishment. If the child is losing his or her temper or becoming frustrated, ask the child to sit in a quiet place for a few minutes without distractions.

Withholding Privileges
This technique involved removing a privilege when the child misbehaves and should be reserved for behaviors that are dangerous or very troublesome.

Token Economy
A token economy involves earning points for positive behavior and losing points for negative behavior. At the end of an agreed upon time, the child may receive a prize

Behavior therapy is a vital part of treatment for ADHD, but it is most effective when collaboration exists between the therapist and the prescriber. It is intended to teach children behavioral, social, and academic skills that are useful in managing ADHD symptoms throughout life. It can improve ADHD symptoms as well as the child's relationship with peers and family members. Medication addresses ADHD on the neurological level to regulate the brain and may be effective in reducing impulsivity and inattention, but it generally doesn't result in the child learning positive behaviors to substitute for the negative ones. For example, the medication may effectively prevent the child from hitting his younger sibling, but it will not teach him what to do instead of hitting. Behavior therapy provides positive alternative behaviors to use.

Behavior therapy, or parent training, can also be beneficial for the parents of children with ADHD. During these sessions, parents learn techniques that can be used to motivate children to change negative behaviors. Parents are taught to set specific, simple, and clear goals for their children. Achievement of these goals is reinforced by a reward system, positive reinforcement, time-outs, withholding privileges, or a token economy. In addition, therapists help parents understand what influences their children's behavior and how to adjust their parenting accordingly to more effectively motivate and reinforce positive behaviors.

One caution about parent behavior training is that the parent shouldn't feel that their current style of parenting is the cause of the child's problems. Instead, it should be considered adaptive parenting, where you are simply using a different approach based on your child's needs. We all have a different approach to parenting. The therapist's goal is to help you discover the style that your child will most positively respond to. Parent training may include

- *Establishing routines.* Structured routines help children feel safe and in control. Please refer to the sample daily routine below. If interested, you may download a free printable sample daily routine from http://authorscott.com/sampledailyroutinechecklistadhd/.
- *Creating clear and consistent expectations and consequences.* Children with ADHD have less control over impulsive behavior and require clear and consistent expectations and consequences to help them understand what is acceptable and what is not.

- *Positive parenting.* Positive statements and parenting helps preserve a child's self-esteem and establishes self-confidence.
- *Maintaining calm.* Children with ADHD tend to be more in tune with their parent's mood state and to mirror what they see. They will detect nonverbal cues—body language, tone of voice, etc.—and often adapt their behavior and mood to that of their parents. If you maintain your calm, they are more likely to maintain their calm.
- *Reinforcing talents.* Some children with ADHD may feel they lack talents, skills, and feel undervalued. Parents play a vital role in helping their children identify and cultivate talents, special abilities, and skills that will help them feel more valuable.

Sample Daily Routine—School Age Children:
This sample daily routine is meant to be a guide to help you establish structure and a predictable daily routine for your child with ADHD. It is best to put the routine in writing (clear and brief wording) in a conspicuous place for your child to refer to and follow. Don't throw in the towel after a few days or even a few weeks just because the routine isn't "working." You need to help your child with ADHD understand that this is not a temporary adjustment, but a permanent way of life that will help him be more successful. Many children with ADHD need incremental time warnings, so you may want to use phrases like "you have five more minutes . . ." If you are committed, firm, and patient (you may need to teach the routine over and over until they do it out of habit) establishing a regular routine can help improve efficiency, make daily activities more manageable, reduce overall family stress, and strengthen family relationships.

7:00 a.m.   **WAKE UP**
Stick with the same wake-up time every day, even on weekends, to make mornings easier and encourage a natural circadian rhythm. Wake

younger children with a gentle touch. Older children can use an alarm. If your child wakes up before the designated time allow him to play in his room quietly without any screen time. As a visual reminder of when he is permitted to get up, consider a dual-color nightlight (available online at places like Amazon.com) that turns green when it is okay to wake up the parents.

7:05 a.m.   **MORNING HYGIENE**

Post a checklist that includes the steps to get ready for the day, such as "make your bed, put on clean clothes, wash face, and brush hair." It may be helpful to organize outfits (underwear, top, bottom, and socks) in a closet organizer identified by the days of the week (Sunday through Saturday). Allowing a child to help pick out his weekly outfits at the beginning of the week can help reduce the struggles of selecting an outfit in the morning or pulling out everything in the dresser to find his favorite Avengers t-shirt.

7:20 a.m.   **BREAKFAST**

Offer two choices of healthy breakfast (with complex carbohydrates and high-quality protein). For, example "Choice number one for breakfast is ____; and choice number two for breakfast is ____." Avoid the "trigger" ingredients like refined sugar, food colorings, and additives. Don't forget any dietary supplements he takes in the morning.

7:40 a.m.   **BRUSH TEETH**

Consider brushing your teeth together, which can help keep him on task and ensure good hygiene.

7:45 a.m.   **EXIT—PUT ON SHOES**

Keep backpack, shoes, and other outdoor gear by the door. Get shoes on (and a jacket and hat if necessary for weather conditions).

7:50 a.m.   **TRAVEL TO SCHOOL**

8:00 a.m. –   **SCHOOL**
2:50 p.m.

2:50 p.m.   **TRAVEL HOME / ENTRANCE**
Ask about your child's day as you travel home. Hang up and put away all outside gear, shoes, and backpack by the door.

3:00 p.m.   **SNACK**
Provide a healthy snack and let your child unwind after school. Children with ADHD often do well eating smaller, more frequent meals and snacks.

3:20 p.m.   **HOMEWORK OR CHORES**
HOMEWORK: Establish a "homework area" where your child consistently sits (or stands) to do his homework. Have all the tools (pen or pencil, calculator, paper, etc.) ready and available in the homework area. Go through your child's backpack together and identify any homework, assignments, or notes that need to be taken care of. Reduce distractions in the homework area (TV, phone calls, activity, unnecessary noise). Play classical music for part of the homework time if desired. Be available to help your child with homework, answer questions, and supervise breaks (stretch, drink, jog in place, etc.). Some children may not be able to sustain their attention on homework for a continuous thirty minutes. Set a timer for 5, 10, or 15 minutes (age appropriate) for 2-minute

active breaks (dancing, jumping jacks, etc.). Praise your child when he puts forth his best effort and finishes required tasks. Waiting until the evening may create a battle, so after a snack is ideal. Set a specific amount of time to complete homework and then stop working on it.

CHORES: If your child has no homework or it is a day off from school, choose appropriate and specific tasks to complete as chores. Consider creating a weekly chore chart to establish consistency and a pattern of chores each day.

3:50 p.m.   **REVIEW HOMEWORK OR CHORES**
Review your child's homework and calmly explain anything he needs to correct. Make sure to praise him for good work or efforts.

4:00 p.m.   **FREE TIME**
Providing free play for activities such as outside play, sports, or other physical activity is as important as structured time. This could even include some limited screen time. However, the American Academy of Pediatrics urges parents to avoid TV viewing for children under age 2 and limit screen time to one or two hours daily for older children. Other experts suggest older children get no more than 1.5 hours of screen time daily—with a 1-hour limit even better. Perhaps a better option than screen time is to play with your child. Play-based interventions can improve ADHD symptoms and nurture a healthier parent-child relationship.

5:30 p.m.   **DINNER PREPARATION**
Enlist the help of your child with age-appropriate dinner preparation steps (setting the table, making the salad, etc.). Giving them specific

tasks to prepare for dinner helps establish a sense of responsibility.

6:00 p.m.   DINNER
Serve a well-balanced meal. Engage your child and the rest of the family in conversation.

6:30 p.m.   DINNER CLEAN UP
Involve your child in dinner age-appropriate dinner clean up (clear the table, put away left overs, load the dishwasher, or dry dishes.

7:00 p.m.   RELAXATION
After dinner should be a time for relaxing and winding down. This is a great time to read with your child or listen to calm music. If TV or a movie is watched, choose shows that are calm, not action thrillers or dramas. Avoid energizing activities like video games or active play. Play a board or card game, color together, draw pictures, or another activity that will promote a more relaxed state to get ready for bed. A 5- to 10-minute deep pressure (deeper or more pressure than a typical light massage) essential oil massage to the back and/or feet using essential oils carefully selected from Chapter 5 can be beneficial and calming.

8:00 p.m.   EVENING SNACK
Allow your child to graze on healthy snacks when he may be hungriest (right before bed).

8:10 p.m.   GET READY FOR BED
Create a detailed checklist of the activities your child should do to get ready for bed (shower or bathe, brush teeth, put on pajamas, put dirty clothes in the laundry hamper, and go to the bathroom).

8:30 p.m.   BEDTIME
Maintain a regular sleep schedule and consistent bedtime. Tuck your child in while singing a calming song, complimenting him on his successes that day, or whatever habitual bedtime routine you follow.

Parents and health professionals would be remiss to dismiss behavior therapy in the management of ADHD. Experience suggests that if children are put on medications first, they are highly unlikely ever to try behavior therapy. Scientists have also discovered that parents who use behavior therapy as an option experience fewer significant problems with their children, and teachers report improved classroom behavior.[205,206,207] With minimal risk to behavior therapy, it is certainly worth a try, and may have better results in the long run than medications alone.

Medications

Medication may help control some ADHD symptoms, but like all medications, there are side effects and risks associated with them. It should also be noted that medication is not the only treatment option, and many parents and children successfully manage ADHD without them. ADHD medications may help improve concentration, reduce impulsivity, and increase planning skills, but they are not a magic pill that will fix all problems associated with ADHD. Even if the medication works, a child may still struggle with relationships—both peer and family, emotional problems, forgetfulness, and absent-mindedness. Unfortunately, many children receive stimulant drugs without behavior therapy, which will not fully address all of the symptoms the child is experiencing. In addition, medications affect children differently, meaning what works for one child may not work—or cause adverse effects—in another child. Several medications are currently approved to treat ADHD, including stimulants and nonstimulants. ADHD medications must be closely controlled and monitored to increase their effectiveness and reduce risks.

Stimulant Medications

Stimulant medications are the most commonly prescribed and widely used medications for ADHD. They have the longest track record and tend to work more rapidly than nonstimulants. Stimulants come in short-acting (taken two to three times per day) and long-acting dosages (taken once per day and last up to twelve hours). These medications work by increasing dopamine—a neurotransmitter associated with pleasure, attention, and movement—and/or norepinephrine levels in the brain. Children with the inattentive subtype of ADHD generally have lower levels of norepinephrine levels, whereas low dopamine levels are commonly found in children with the hyperactive-impulsive subtype of ADHD. For many people, stimulant medications enhance attention and focus while reducing hyperactivity and impulsiveness.[208,209]

Different types of stimulant medications exist:

- Methylphenidate (Concerta, Daytrana, Metadate, Ritalin) stimulants are often the first choice for treating ADHD. These drugs work by stimulating the central nervous system and increasing dopamine and norepinephrine levels in the brain—typically about an hour after the medication is taken.[210] Interestingly, scientists were baffled as to why methylphenidate worked for ADHD until they studied addictive drugs like cocaine. That is because methylphenidate works in the brain similarly to cocaine—it blocks cells from disposing of dopamine, which increases dopamine levels in the brain. Dopamine helps control behavior, so having optimum levels of it in the brain is important for ADHD. They can be habit-forming and should only be taken according to instructions.
- Amphetamine-based stimulants (Adderall, Dexedrine, Dextrostat) also stimulate the central nervous system and influence levels of dopamine and norepinephrine.

Studies suggest that amphetamines increase norepinephrine levels significantly more than methylphenidate stimulants.[211] They also have a longer half-life (the time it takes the body to metabolize half of a substance, whereupon the action of the substance is reduced from its initial effectiveness) than methylphenidate (four to six hours compared to two to three hours), suggesting the clinical effect is more long-lasting.[212]

- Methamphetamine hydrochloride (Desoxyn) is also a central nervous system stimulant and believed to influence dopamine and norepinephrine levels in the brain. Methamphetamine hydrochloride triggers the fight-or-flight response, which releases stress hormones, elevates heart rate and blood pressure, and restricts blood flow to muscles away from the gut. In the short term these drugs increase alertness, but this is followed by a crash that can leave the person feeling irritable, extremely exhausted, and depressed. It is highly addictive in nature and lasts longer in the body than Adderall, so it typically is only prescribed when other medications are ineffective.

- Dextromethylphenidate hydrochloride (Focalin) is a stimulant similar to methylphenidate (methylphenidate is actually a mixture of dexmethylphenidate and levomethylphenidate). It is believed to increase both dopamine and norepinephrine levels in the brain. An extended release (Focalin XR) form delivers half of the medication as an immediate dose, with the other half is released later to provide longer-lasting symptom relief and reduce the side effects.

- Lisdexamfetamine dimesylate (Vyvanse) is a stimulant medication that is actually a therapeutically inactive prodrug. A prodrug is a substance that must be converted to another substance to be effective. The body must convert the lisdexamfetamine dimesylate to a more therapeutically active form before it has a clinical effect. Like all ADHD stimulants, it is believed to increase the availability of dopamine and norepinephrine in the brain. The manufacturer of Vyvanse, Shire Pharmaceuticals, claims that because the drug is released over an extended period of time, it is less prone to dependence and abuse.

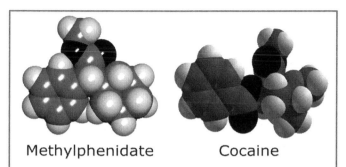

Methylphenidate   Cocaine

Both methylphenidate and cocaine are powerful stimulants that increase dopamine levels in the brain. The molecular structure of both is strikingly similar, and they act much alike (entering the brain at similar rates, and targeting similar brain regions). Methylphenidate is only less addictive because of its administration method and the fact that cocaine has a higher dissipation rate (requiring its use more often to maintain a high). Cocaine is snorted or injected, allowing it to flood the brain quickly. On the other hand, methylphenidate is taken orally, so it takes longer to reach the brain.

Many parents wonder why stimulants may affect ADHD symptoms. It doesn't seem logical to give a child who is already hyperactive a stimulant. However, this can be explained by the fact that children with ADHD are constantly self-stimulating. To satisfy their need for stimulation they wiggle, fidget, talk, or perform other stimulating activities. By providing stimulation through a medication, they no longer have the urge to self-stimulate.

Stimulant medications are frequently abused for their ability to suppress appetite, encourage weight loss, boost concentration and focus, and enhance performance.[213] Abuse of stimulant medications for a "high" or to improve grades is growing among teenagers and young adults.[214] Some teens and adults hold a belief that stimulants will make them smarter and enhance their performance in school, but research suggests this is not the case. In fact, studies report that students who abuse prescription stimulants actually have lower GPAs in high school and college, skip class more often, and experience cognitive deficits when compared to students who do not abuse the drugs.[215,216] Unfortunately, it is probable that a person who takes ADHD medications as a mental-performance-enhancing drug will experience increased mental focus and a drive to get things done. Because of this, "study drugs" are passed around on campuses like candy. The practice of abusing stimulants for better grades in school is a serious concern with dire consequences. A number of health consequences may be the result of a temporary increase in focus: dependence, addiction, an exhaustion crash, depression, anxiety, cardiovascular risks, and insomnia; not to mention the legal risks: fines, jail time, and suspension or expulsion from school.

Risks are a possibility even among children for whom these drugs are prescribed. Beyond the abuse potential of stimulants, they also have many side effects and risks, some serious. Misuse of stimulants is particularly concerning and can cause serious side effects such as psychosis, heart attack, cardiomyopathy (disease of the heart muscle), and even sudden death.[217] Other side effects include restlessness, nervousness, difficulty sleeping, headache, irritability, mood swings, dizziness, tics, rapid heartbeat, upset stomach, loss of appetite, and depression. Statistics show that almost half of people who take ADHD medications experience at least one side effect, the most common being loss of appetite, difficulty sleeping, and mood swings.[218] Studies suggest that 8 to 9 percent of people treated with stimulants also experience tics or involuntary muscle movements.[219,220] Careful monitoring of the drugs and their appropriate use must be a priority to reduce risks, both short- and long-term.

Some additional safety concerns associated with ADHD stimulant medications include unknown neurological effects, cardiovascular risks, and psychiatric disorders. The long-term effects of stimulants on the brain are not yet fully understood.

Some scientists have observed that dopamine receptors in the brain have increased in response to medication, which suggests that a tolerance could be built-up over time. Studies have shown that stimulants have a very small increased risk of adverse cardiovascular system events, including increased blood pressure, rapid heart rate, and sudden cardiac death.[221,222] Children with existing heart problems are more susceptible to these adverse effects. It is possible that stimulant medications could trigger or exacerbate psychiatric problems such as anxiety, depression, paranoia, aggression, and hostility.[223] Those with a family history of psychiatric disorders should be closely monitored when taking stimulants.[224] All of this makes it critical that a thorough family and medical history be conducted by a qualified physician before medications are prescribed. In reality, the most qualified person to make this diagnosis may be a psychiatrist that has attended medical school and trained in general medicine in addition to psychotherapy.

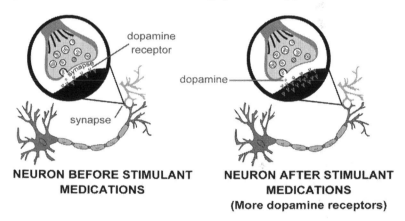

dopamine receptor

dopamine

synapse

NEURON BEFORE STIMULANT MEDICATIONS

NEURON AFTER STIMULANT MEDICATIONS
(More dopamine receptors)

Nonstimulant Medications

Nonstimulant medications were approved for the treatment of ADHD in 2003, so they are relatively new to the ADHD medication realm. Some physicians believe there is not enough evidence to support their efficacy currently. Nonstimulants are primarily used as a "last resort" medication when stimulants haven't worked or have caused intolerable side effects. Additional reasons to choose a nonstimulant medications include comorbid (the presence of more than one disorder) psychiatric disorder, concern for stimulant abuse, and medical problems that make stimulant use difficult.

There are several nonstimulant medications prescribed to treat ADHD, some of which are antidepressants:

- Atomoxetine hydrochloride (Strattera) was first developed as an antidepressant, but when studies showed it was not effective for depression, it was tried for ADHD. It works by increasing norepinephrine availability in the brain and is considered a selective norepinephrine reuptake inhibitor (SNRI). Norepinephrine affects the part of the brain involved in attention and impulsivity control, so influencing its availability to the brain may reduce ADHD symptoms. Because it is a nonstimulant, it can take up to four weeks to work.

- Guanfacine (Intuniv) works on symptoms of ADHD that stimulants are not very effective for—emotional imbalance, social aggressiveness, and hyperarousal. It is often used in combination with stimulant medications for this reason. Guanfacine works by stimulating alpha-2 adrenergic receptors in the nervous system (called an alpha-2-adrenergic agonist), which causes a decrease in sympathetic nervous system activity. Decreased sympathetic nervous system activity has a calming effect that reduces stress, blood pressure, and adrenaline levels. Guanfacine is believed to help regulate norepinephrine release as well.

- Clonidine hydrochloride (Kapvay) is also an alpha-2-adrenergic agonist, which works by decreasing sympathetic nervous system activity. It is often taken in combination with stimulant medication, but research suggests that doing so may increase the risk of side effects, particularly drowsiness.[225] Some physicians are concerned about how alpha-2-adrenergic agonist drugs will affect blood pressure because their primary use is for high blood pressure.

- Nortriptyline hydrochloride (Pamelor) is a tricyclic antidepressant that increases serotonin and norepinephrine availability in the brain. It does not influence dopamine availability. It may be a good option for those who have failed to respond to previous medications. A clinical trial found that 76 percent of people who failed to respond to an average of four previous medications experienced moderate to significant relief of ADHD symptoms with nortriptyline hydrochloride.[226] Clinical effects take from a few days to a few weeks to achieve. It is important that an electrocardiogram (EKG) be performed before beginning a tricyclic antidepressant and the heart is continually monitored during treatment because of certain cardiovascular risks.
- Imipramine hydrochloride (Tofranil) is also a tricyclic antidepressant that has been extensively studied for treating ADHD.[227] Like other tricyclic antidepressants, it increases serotonin and norepinephrine availability in the brain. It typically takes two to four weeks to experience benefits. Imipramine seems to be most effective in people with the inattentive subtypes of ADHD.
- Desipramine hydrochloride (Norpramin) is a tricyclic antidepressant that increases norepinephrine and to a minor extent serotonin levels in the brain. It also blocks parasympathetic nervous system activity—the division of the nervous system involved in sexual arousal, salivation, urination, digestion, and defecation.[228] It usually takes about two to four weeks to produce results. Many clinicians are hesitant to prescribe desipramine because of cases reporting sudden death in children who were taking the drug.[229] Imipramine and nortriptyline are far more likely to be prescribed if tricyclic antidepressant therapy is used for ADHD.
- Nontricyclic antidepressants are also sometimes used for ADHD. Common nontricyclic antidepressants used for this purpose include bupropion (Wellbutrin, Buproban,

Aplenzin, Budeprion, Zyban), venlafaxine, and atomoxetine. These drugs influence the availability of serotonin and norepinephrine in the brain and may be used if depression exists with the ADHD (comorbidity).

SIDE EFFECTS OF NONSTIMULANTS	
Strattera	Decreased appetite, nausea, vomiting, fatigue, indigestion, dizziness, mood swings, belching, irregular menstruation, cough, difficulty urinating, headache, heartburn, irritability, sexual dysfunction, pain or tenderness around the eyes or cheekbones, shortness of breath, insomnia, dry mouth
Intuniv	Blurred vision, sweating, weakness, fatigue, confusion, dizziness, lightheadedness when standing, difficulty breathing, cough, increased urination, irregular heartbeat, chest pain, tightness in chest
Kapvay	Drowsiness, nausea, constipation, headache, fatigue, irritability, diarrhea, excessive thirst, tremors, anxiety, nightmares, insomnia, sore throat, elevated body temperature, sexual dysfunction, darkening of the skin, loss of appetite, dry, itching or burning eyes
Pamelor	Drowsiness, dizziness, insomnia, nausea, rash, blurred vision, constipation, cramps, high or low blood pressure, abnormal heart rate, liver or kidney toxicity, photosensitivity, hair loss, diarrhea, sexual dysfunction, seizures, delirium, delusions, tremors, fatigue, indigestion
Tofranil	Abdominal pain, blurred vision, irregular heartbeat, tingling feelings, chest pain, confusion, cough, urinary difficulties, dizziness, delusions, fever, fatigue, weakness, hostility, irritability, loss of balance or coordination, nightmares, slow speech, seizures, swelling, uncontrolled movements, yellow eyes or skin

Norpramin	Drowsiness, blurred vision, insomnia, dizziness, hair loss, diarrhea, rash, high or low blood pressure, weakness, irregular heartbeat, delusions, liver or kidney toxicity, high or low blood sugar, nausea, anxiety, fatigue, acid reflux, constipation
Wellbutrin	Agitation, headache, nausea, stomachache, vision problems, constipation, dizziness, ringing in ears, sore throat, rash, itching, muscle aches, tremors, decreased libido, irregular heartbeat, hyperventilation, insomnia, irritability, shortness of breath

One factor to consider when determining whether medication is an appropriate or feasible option is compliance. Will the child take the medication as prescribed, and will this compliance continue through adolescence and the teen years? It is typically around adolescence or the early teen years when children begin to express autonomy and challenge their parents. This may lead to noncompliance in taking ADHD medications. In addition, studies show that ADHD changes over time, and about 65 percent of children experience full or partial remission by age 25.[230,231] Study data indicates that the requirement for medication may actually decline over time as the child ages. The third factor in compliance is the fact that the liver changes as the child grows, which may modify the metabolism of medications and change the way these medications act on the child. They may feel different or experience personality changes requiring adjustments in the dosage of their medication. The short of it is, if the child will not continue to take medication as prescribed, managing ADHD symptoms through medication will be very difficult.

If you decide to discontinue ADHD medication, do not do so without your health professional's approval and guidance. Because the medications alter the availability of vital neurotransmitters, a sudden change (such as discontinuing medication cold turkey) may cause headache, depression, fatigue, mood alterations, unusual behavior, and changes in heartbeat. Here are a few practical tips to discontinue ADHD medications in collaboration with your health professional:

1. *Work with your doctor.* This bears repeating because you need to report any problems experienced while quitting the medication as soon as they occur, not when it has become an emergency.
2. *Reduce the medication gradually.* Don't abruptly stop taking the medication unless you are advised to by your physician. A better approach is to half the medication for a week or so and monitor behavior and symptoms before reducing the remaining medication dosage.
3. *Choose the right time to reduce medication.* It's best not to reduce ADHD medication during periods of stress or major life changes. For example, a freshman in college with ADHD wouldn't want to quit her medication during finals week. Similarly, it may be best for an elementary-age child to reduce medication over the summer when there is less risk of disrupting school.
4. *Find a therapist or counselor.* It makes sense to learn coping strategies and ways to structure life to help manage symptoms. A counselor or therapist can provide tips and tools that will help you better cope with a life without medication.

As with all medications, a decision to use or not to use certain medications should be jointly made with the patient, parents, and health professional. Although a large number of children with ADHD will benefit from medication, some don't need to take it, and up to 30 percent of children do not experience significant benefits. It all boils down to weighing the risks versus the benefits of medication.

Making School Successful for the Child with ADHD

One of the greatest challenges for the child with ADHD is the restrictive requirements of the school environment. Children's very nature of being energetic, talkative, distracted, and outgoing is in stark contrast to the expected behavior of the textbook student. Indeed, children with ADHD may try their hardest to avoid fidgeting and disrupting class, but this only bottles up their need for stimulation and may lead to an explosive outburst. To reduce serious problems in school, parents and teachers should take charge of ADHD by making a few simple but valuable modifications and accommodations.

Today's school setting requires children to sit still, listen quietly, pay attention, and concentrate on assignments—all things that children with ADHD struggle with frequently. Children with ADHD are often disruptive, hyperactive, and inattentive at school—behaviors that take away from instruction time, disrupt others in the class, and quickly frustrate a teacher. Teachers of children with ADHD—which, given the numbers of children diagnosed with ADHD, should include all teachers—should understand that these children are willing to learn; their brains just get in the way. Skilled teachers know how to adapt their teaching for all students in their classrooms, including children with ADHD. So the question is, how do you ensure your child gets in that teacher's class?

Choosing the "Perfect" School and Teacher

The first step to ensuring your child gets a teacher accomplished at adjusting her teaching approach to children with ADHD is to research, research, and research some more. This involves talking to neighbors, friends, parents of current students, and other connections about the school and teachers. In addition, check out the school and district's website. Review their mission statement and goals, review the principal and teachers' available information, and consider calling them or sending an e-mail to help determine if the school and teacher are the right fit. This research could be the difference between a miserable and frustrating school year and one that goes smoothly and fosters a learning environment that your child can thrive in.

School administrators have the daunting task of leading a school of unique students, diverse teachers, and assorted staff, with a limited budget, and then they're expected to maximize student success, growth, and achievement. They are not likely to respond well to demanding parents who order them to place their child in Mrs. Perfect's class. Instead, parents should meet with the school administrator to describe the qualities and characteristics that Mrs. Perfect possesses that will help their child excel in school. For example, you may share with the administrator that you are looking for the following qualities in a teacher: provides structure and routine, firmness, kindness, understanding, and a strict-yet-gentle approach. If the administrator asks for a teacher's name that fits these qualities, now is your opportunity to recommend the teacher you want. Be sure to thank the administrator for his or her time after the visit. This short conversation may land you the skilled teacher that will allow your child to thrive in the coming school year.

Once a teacher has been selected with the help of the administrator, your next task is to meet with Mrs. Perfect before the school year starts. Explain the reason for your appointment request when you make the appointment—that you want to discuss ways you can partner with the teacher to make your child's school year as successful as possible. Most teachers will appreciate your willingness to be involved. Back to school night is not the appropriate time to have this conversation. You need to do this when adequate time is available and both you and the teacher are prepared to have a productive discussion. During this meeting, the following should be discussed:

- what informal interventions have worked for your child in the past;
- your desire to partner with the teacher and your willingness to help;
- mutually agreed upon expectations;
- the individual strengths and needs of your child; and
- teaching and disciplinary methods, such as how to intervene when your child is disruptive, how positive behavior and quality work will be reinforced, and what interventions can be incorporated to make learning easier for your child.

Parent-Teacher Communication

Daily communication between parents and the school is vital for the success of all students. It is even more important for the parents of children with ADHD, and allows parents to monitor their child's progress. If your school has an agenda, review it carefully with your child. The primary purpose of the agenda is to help students stay organized and keep track of assignments and homework on a daily basis. Keep in mind our previous discussion on how the brains of children with ADHD are often different. Irregularities in synaptic firing among children with ADHD leads to your child hearing half of what is shared and understanding about one-third. The agenda will not be a one-and-done situation. Instead, parents should be aware that they will need to reteach the agenda multiple times.

Parents may also request a daily note or brief report of their child's performance. The teacher can create this report that includes homework requirements, behavior, and accomplishments for the day. Remember, though: if you request the report, you must read it and respond appropriately. Help your child understand that this report is not a punishment but a means of facilitating effective communication. Impress upon your child that both you and the teacher care about him or her and want to ensure his or her school efforts are properly recognized. Calmly communicate any defeats and celebrate the success reported by the teacher in this communication. Consider a small reward for positive behaviors or goal accomplishments identified by the teacher. This may seem like a lot to do, but it may be the difference between a child's success or defeat when it comes to education.

Organizing Backpacks

An organized and maintained backpack can be one the greatest supports of a child with ADHD. Instead of being a bottomless pit of lost papers, school supplies, and important information, an organized backpack is a systemized portable receptacle for school essentials. Keep the backpack in a designated spot at home. This can avoid hunting for the backpack that may have been left in the car, under the bed, or another obscure hiding place. Purchase a backpack with multiple compartments to keep all of your child's supplies and notes close at hand. Items to consider including in the back pack include an agenda, reasonable supplies, folders for KEEP HOME and RETURN TO SCHOOL, and color-coded folders for each subject (i.e., green for science, blue for math, red for English, etc.). A daily routine of reviewing the contents of the backpack with your child should be established.

Fostering Friendship and Positive Peer Relationships at School and Home

Sometimes children with ADHD struggle with friendships and need help keeping friends. This is mainly due to children with ADHD not fully understanding how they are perceived by their peers. They may commit social blunders, offend friends, struggle with taking turns, make thoughtless comments, or become overly aggressive during play. All of this can damage friendships and peer relationships without the ADHD child even understanding why. Parents can be huge advocates to help children develop better social skills and sustain satisfying friendships and positive peer relationships. Consider these tips to help your child with ADHD make and keep friends:

- Model, demonstrate, and rehearse proper social skills with your child. One area to particularly model is how to use positive instead of harsh language. Teach your child to say, "How about we play soccer?" instead of "That's a stupid game."
- Coach your child about what makes a good friend and how the child should behave while with other children. Include manners (how to approach other children appropriately, sharing, asking permission, etc.), ways to handle frustration and anger (counting to ten before reacting, ways to cool down before choosing a course of action, etc.), and acceptable way to resolve conflict (talking instead of using physical contact, asking for adult assistance, etc.).
- Ask your school counselor if there is a social group your child can participate in. If not, look for an afterschool group, like the YMCA, 4-H Afterschool, AmeriCorps, Scouts, or church groups.
- Consider younger children as friends first. Children with ADHD often lag behind their peers in social skills and tend to be more immature. Connecting your child with a younger peer will allow him or her to master his or her social skills without being ridiculed.

- Invite a few of your child's peers over to your home where play can occur in a more comfortable and familiar environment. It also allows you the chance to observe his or her interactions and coach better social skills when necessary.
- Lastly, register your child for a social-skills program such as Project ACHIEVE's Stop & Think Social Skills Program. It never hurts to have your child hear these social-skills tips from another person to reinforce what you are sharing.

School Accommodations and Interventions

If informal interventions are unfruitful for whatever reason, it may be time to seek a more formalized plan for your child. Two formalized plans to advocate for your struggling child include an Individualized Education Plan (IEP) and 504 Plan. Public schools are required to create an IEP for every child receiving special education services (educational services tailored to meet the needs of students based on a disability or learning difficulty). An IEP plan is a written document meant to address each child's unique learning issues and develop educational goals. A 504 Plan provides services and changes to the learning environment to meet the needs of the child as adequately as other students. Formalized evaluations must be administered for your child to receive either an IEP or 504 Plan. Federal law mandates both plans, but the evaluation process will differ by state and school district. Ideally, you should make an appointment with the school counselor or psychologist to determine the IEP/504 Plan process for your school.

The process of securing accommodations for a child with ADHD can be intimidating and demanding. To be eligible for an IEP, your child must have one or more of the thirteen specific disabilities listed in the Individuals with Disabilities Education Act (IDEA); and that disability must affect your child's educational performance or ability to learn from the general curriculum. If your child does not qualify for an IEP, he or she may be eligible for a 504 Plan. To be eligible for a 504 Plan, your child must have a documented, long-term physical or mental impairment that substantially limits one or more life activities (i.e., reading or concentrating). Some organizations exist that provide special advocates that represent your child's interests to receive reasonable adaptations as well. They can be very helpful in facilitating cooperation, coordination, and the exchange of information between the school and parents. Document your child's difficulties, be assertive, and resolutely request reasonable changes that will enrich your child's learning opportunities and ability to succeed in school.

Thirteen IDEA Disabilities

1. Specific learning disability (dyslexia, auditory processing disorder, etc.)
2. Other health impairment (limits child's strength, energy, or alertness)
3. Autism spectrum disorder
4. Emotional disturbance (anxiety, bipolar disorder, depression, etc.)
5. Speech or language impairment
6. Visual impairment, including blindness
7. Deafness
8. Hearing impairment (hearing loss not covered by deafness)
9. Deaf-blindness (both hearing and visual impairments)
10. Orthopedic impairment (impairment to a child's body, i.e. cerebral palsy)
11. Intellectual disability
12. Traumatic brain injury
13. Multiple disabilities (one or more of the above conditions)

Tips for Educational Professionals to Enhance Learning Among Children with ADHD

Teachers and school administrators must tailor their teaching to each child's individual needs and strengths. Things to consider include teaching methods, how to intervene when disruptive behaviors occur, how to reinforce positive behavior or quality work, and what accommodations can be made to make learning easier for children with ADHD. This won't be easy and will require great patience, creativity, consistency, and, most of all, a positive attitude.

Ideas to improve interactions with and the educational experience of children with ADHD include:

- Seat them at the front of the classroom near the teacher and away from distractions.
- Praise the child's behavior or hard work in public, but only discuss negative behavior in private.
- Consider placing children who are well-behaved role models to his or her left and right.
- Allow him or her extra time to complete assignments and consider breaking larger projects into smaller, bite-sized pieces (i.e., fold assignment papers in half).
- Combine written instructions with oral instructions.
- Ask him or her questions to engage him or her in lessons.
- Create a private signal that can cue him or her to stay on task.
- As difficult as it may be, ignore minor negative behavior.
- Allow him or her to play with paperclips, doodle on paper, or another stimulating but less disruptive behavior.
- Capture the attention of the daydreamer with a phrase such as "one, two, three, eyes on me."
- Involve him or her in physical activity such as handing out papers, running errands, or cleaning the chalkboard.
- Assign him or her special responsibilities or a leadership role in the classroom—this may be important to improve peer relationships.
- Be very cautious about taking away recess as a punishment. Children with ADHD need to run, play, and release built-up energy.

Leveling the Playing Field at Recess

Now that you have advocated for reasonable accommodations in the classroom, the playground must be considered. Any child can become a victim of bullying or exclusion, but children with

ADHD are at greater risk. They may appear awkward to their peers and stand out because of their impulsivity, inappropriate behavior, hyperactivity, or intensity. Based on observations of this behavior by their peers, they may garner the attention of a bully who thrives on extreme emotional responses, or be excluded because they are different. No child should have to spend a day at school feeling afraid, humiliated, or nervous because of bullying, or feel unhappy and unwanted because they are left out. In addition, this heightened state of alert, stress, emotional imbalance, and worry over bullying and exclusion can be harmful to your child's school performance and behavior at home. Fortunately, strategies exist to protect your child from the damaging effects of bullying and exclusion that will help him or her have a better playground experience.

- Teach your child to enter an ongoing activity with "May I play?" or "May I join you?" If the answer is no, teach him or her to move on to another group rather than lash out.
- If your child reports bullying to you, praise him or her for being willing to come forward. Listen to his or her feelings and encourage him or her to be honest about his or her actions and reactions to the bullying. Document all the details and a timeline of events, including any witnesses.
- If the bullying is of a serious nature, contact the teacher first, followed by the counselor, principal, and district if necessary. Share with them all the details and strategize together what can be done to improve the situation. Parents are strongly advised to tell school administrators and teachers that you don't want peer mediation (putting the victim and bully in the same room to work it out), which may further traumatize your child and intensify the bullying.
- Explain how bullies work (a child may bully because of low self-esteem, lack of attention, or abuse at home) and without blaming how some of your child's behavior (talking too much, blurting out inappropriate remarks, misbehaving, etc.) may draw the negative attention of a bully. Help your child learn how to keep a low profile

(quieter voice, thinking before speaking, etc.) to avoid problems.

- Teach them to avoid telling on the bully every time it occurs. Instead, encourage them to go stand by the playground monitor or teacher and say, "Billy is picking on me, so I'd like to stand by you instead of getting in trouble."
- Create positive social experiences for your child with other children. Invite a few peers over to do something your child really enjoys.
- Most importantly, show your child that you love him or her and reinforce that he or she is special and wonderful no matter what the bully says or does.

Every child deserves an equal opportunity to have a rewarding and positive educational experience. Without this equal chance for a rewarding education, you may never know what your child could have accomplished. Parents have the primary responsibility for the care and nurture of their children, but most teachers are eager to partner with you in ensuring your child receives the best educational experience possible. Be an advocate for your child and collect partners (teachers, administrators, counselors, etc.) to give your child the best chance for success. Remember: there is no such thing as "fair." Whether it's interventions, an IEP or 504 plan, or other reasonable accommodations, it is all about leveling the playing field so that all can access education equally.

Conclusion

There is more than one option to manage ADHD, and all options that have a chance of effectiveness should be considered, with a preference for the least invasive and least harmful option. Don't overlook the benefits of behavior therapy. It may be the only thing required to see improvements in your child. If not, medications and complementary options are also available. Educate yourself on all of the options offered to manage ADHD. If a medication is prescribed, ask questions and investigate the risks versus the rewards of the medication. Make school as fun and enjoyable as possible by partnering with the teacher and administration. Be your child's advocate and do your best to provide him or her with equal chances to have a satisfying education. Give your child the best chance of success through reasonable accommodations at school. Be persistent. Be patient. And do your best to help your child.

4

THOUGHTFUL EATING FOR ADHD

Nutrition is the foundation of all health. What we eat is broken down and used by the body, literally becoming part of us. Your body relies on a steady flow of nutrients to work optimally, and this is no different among children with ADHD. While nutrition is far from the only factor or consideration when it comes to ADHD, research does suggest that what a child consumes has a correlation with ADHD symptoms. The majority of scientists largely dismiss the connection between food and ADHD, but parents, savvy clinicians, and some research suggest that eating nutritionally dense foods may improve attentiveness and reduce behavioral problems.[232,233] Although digestion is one of the last things on physicians' and even parents' minds for managing ADHD, mindful nutritional shifts may indeed improve focus and reduce behavioral challenges in some children.

One of the greatest challenges with nutritional strategies and ADHD is that there is no easy way to identify if your child will benefit from a nutritional shift. A variety of foods could possibly hinder or benefit your child's ADHD symptoms. In reality, a nutritional shift takes patience and a lot of trial and error. And you should keep in mind that what works for one child may not necessarily work for another child. Nutritional shifts must be customized to the individual but generally involve four primary strategies:

1. Reduce sugar and refined carbohydrates in favor of high-quality protein.
2. Eliminate or reduce food sensitivities or allergies.
3. Restore optimal levels of nutrients that may be deficient.
4. Rebuild gut health and restore intestinal balance.

Reduce Sugar and Refined Carbohydrates in Favor of High-Quality Protein

One of the most popular nutritional approaches to ADHD is to reduce or eliminate sugar and refined carbohydrates in favor of high-quality protein. Diets high in sugar and refined carbohydrates may contribute to malnourishment and nutritional deficiencies because they are empty calories (high calorie, poor nutrient density, inadequate vitamins and minerals). In addition, too much sugar can lead to disturbances of blood sugar control, cellular responses to insulin, disrupted gut flora, and increase inflammatory responses to metabolism (advanced glycosylation end-products, or AGEs). You can't expect to give your child inadequate nourishment and function at her best.

Some science substantiates this approach because the brain requires protein (amino acids, particularly tyrosine and branched-chain amino acids) to trigger the production of neurotransmitters (dopamine and norepinephrine) involved in alertness.[234,235] On the other hand, carbohydrates trigger the release of neurotransmitters (serotonin release and tryptophan uptake) that cause drowsiness.[236] Hence, food can alter the balance and availability of key neurotransmitters in the brain. Increasing research supports the idea that a nutritional shift in favor of high-quality protein and reduced sugar and refined carbohydrate consumption may reduce ADHD symptoms.

Most research investigating the link between sugar intake and ADHD symptoms has not found a strong link.[237] But these findings may be partly due to the amount of sugar consumed by the average child these days. The average American child these days takes sugar by the teaspoons and tablespoon because of highly sweetened foods. So how can you determine the effect of sugar consistently when lots of sugar is the norm in a typical American diet? Parents who have children with ADHD strongly disagree with studies that say sugar doesn't trigger ADHD symptoms, but scientists say this is largely due to a bias that sugar causes ADHD or aggravates symptoms.[238] Some scientists have connected sugar consumption with ADHD symptoms, including a Yale study that found high-sugar diets may increase inattention in a specific subset of children with ADHD.

Sugar-laden energy drinks and soft drinks also have a controversial relationship with ADHD symptoms. Yale researchers found that children who consume energy drinks (energy drinks are high sugar and high caffeine, so the caffeine may contribute as well) are 66 percent more likely to experience hyperactivity and inattention symptoms.[239] What the researchers reported was that for every sugar-sweetened beverage a teen consumes, his or her risk of hyperactivity and inattention increases by 14 percent. Remarkably, middle school students who drank energy drinks were 66 percent more likely to be hyperactive and inattentive. Energy drinks really should be severely limited in adolescents and teens, and soda should be limited to an occasional beverage.

Recent studies in Australia, Germany, and Norway have also linked soft drink consumption to hyperactivity and inattention.[240,241,242] What researchers observed was that soft drink consumption alters hundreds of proteins in the cortex region of the brain responsible for healthy cellular function, DNA communication, and decision making. This confirmed findings of an earlier study that soda consumption negatively affects learning and memory.[243] These studies have reopened the debate about sugar and its association with ADHD symptoms and, in the very least, suggest some children may be more "sugar sensitive."[244] It certainly is possible that some children are more sensitive to sugar and their symptoms are aggravated more easily by it.

We have all heard that breakfast is the most important meal of the day. It sets the rest of the day up and provides your body much needed nutrients after the "fast" overnight. Indeed, eating breakfast helps children perform better in school (better math and reading scores, improved attention, fewer behavioral problems, and lower depression, anxiety, and hyperactivity).[245,246] For children with ADHD, breakfast matters even more—particularly what is eaten at breakfast. Breakfast should supply wholesome carbohydrates and high-quality protein to start the child's day off right and provide a steady flow of nutrients.

High-quality proteins like eggs, beans, nuts, fish, turkey, chicken, and lean grass-fed beef may help a person with ADHD in a few ways. First, neurons rely on proteins to transmit nerve impulses from the brain that tell the body what to do. Protein must also be supplied to the brain to repair damaged neurons and ensure they function optimally. Second, if you choose to use medications, adequate protein in the diet helps absorb the medicine, which will make it work more quickly. Third, the breakdown products of protein metabolism—amino acids—are vital to the production of tyrosine, which helps produce both dopamine and norepinephrine. Increased availability of these key neurotransmitters helps improve alertness and balance energy levels. Lastly, children with ADHD have lower levels of the amino acid tryptophan and deficiencies in the ability to transport amino acids that are vital to normal brain function and activity.[247] Protein sources such as egg whites, sesame seeds, spirulina, spinach, and fish supply good levels of tryptophan, which is necessary for the production of serotonin. Low serotonin levels may increase impulsivity, aggressive behavior, and decrease sustained attention.[248,249] All of this suggests that getting adequate protein levels from food is vital to the successful management of ADHD symptoms.

Children with ADHD tend to be overstimulated and burn more calories. In addition, medications they take may reduce their appetite. Pairing these two factors may lead to children with ADHD being "hangry" due to hormonal imbalances. The science behind "hangry" is something like this. As you consume nutrients throughout the day, your body distributes them from the bloodstream to organs and tissues and for use as energy. The longer you go between nutrients, the less of these nutrients available for distribution. If your blood-glucose levels fall far enough, your brain sends alarms that it is starving because it is greatly dependent on glucose to function optimally. In addition to the alarm, the brain floods the body with fight-or-flight hormones—including adrenaline and cortisol—that can make someone "hangry." This makes providing sustainable calories like those in protein-rich foods and wholesome carbohydrates critical to help kids feel full longer, reduce surges and collapses in blood-glucose, and prevent the subsequent release of stress hormones.

We have just scratched the surface of what could be said about nutrition for general well-being. The scope of this book is not to define an exact list of foods to eat and not eat, but to share guidelines and suggestions to evaluate. Moreover, we are all biologically unique, which alters what the best foods are for each individual person. To determine an appropriate nutritional plan for your child, please see a holistic nutritionist who can help develop an individualized plan.

After all the debate, it is certainly at least worth a try to eliminate or reduce sugar and refined carbohydrates from the diet and see if it makes a difference. The best way to determine if sugar or refined carbs may in fact be a trigger for your child's ADHD symptoms is to allow him or her to consume sugar for one week. Keep a written log to monitor your child's behavior and symptoms. Remove sugar or refined carbs or both from his or her diet the next week and compare the results. If your child's symptoms are better the second week, ignore what science says and reduce or eliminate sugar or refined carbs or both from his or her diet.

Eliminating or Reducing Food Sensitivities or Allergies

The concept of eliminating foods to improve health began in the 1920s and 1930s when researchers Albert Rowe and C. P. Lapage suggested that diet directly influenced the health of the nervous system.[250,251] Since then, research has discovered that certain foods affect brain electrical activity and, therefore, may influence ADHD symptoms.[252] The purpose of elimination diets is to remove foods that commonly cause allergies or sensitivities (wheat and gluten, corn, soy, dairy, peanuts, seafood, and eggs) that may cause sensitivities or allergies, including artificial ingredients in foods (food dyes, artificial sweeteners, MSG, and preservatives). Elimination diets can eliminate a single food or multiple foods at once. Although just beginning to be understood, ADHD is common among children with food allergies.[253,254] Based on this, the topic is worthy of exploring and gaining a better understanding of.

Elimination diets are usually started by consuming foods that are least likely to cause reactions such as chicken, rice, bananas, apples, cucumbers, carrots, broccoli, cauliflower, and cabbage. If symptoms reduce during this elimination phase (about two weeks), foods are slowly reintroduced into the diet one at a time to see whether they cause a reaction. If no change is observed during the elimination phase of eating, it isn't likely your child will benefit from eliminating specific foods. However, if you notice a difference during the first two weeks it may be helpful to continue the elimination diet and determine what foods may trigger symptoms. This is done by reintroducing one excluded food each day and monitoring your child for changes (more fidgeting, trouble sleeping, etc.). If a reaction is noticed, eliminate the food again. Your child may outgrow the sensitivity, and so you can reintroduce the food a year or so later.

Food colorings are definitely something worth eliminating from the diet. Artificial food dyes (or colorings) affect childhood behavior regardless whether the child has ADHD or not, but those with ADHD seem to be more susceptible to adverse effects.[255] These small synthetic molecules have the ability to bind with proteins in the body, which allows them to avoid detection by the immune system. The immune system is unable to differentiate these molecular hitchhikers from normal proteins, leaving it unable to recognize, defend against, and eliminate food colorings that dysregulate the immune system. In addition, food dyes inhibit the activity of an enzyme (sulfotransferase 1A1) involved in dopamine availability in the brain and play a role in ADHD symptoms.[256] A review of research concluded that up to 89 percent of children with ADHD react to artificial food colors.[257] A buildup of synthetic food colorings can increase inflammation in the body, cause autoimmune disorders, increase intestinal permeability, and trigger brain and behavioral disorders.[258] All of this leads to a cascade of events that may be a trigger for ADHD symptoms.

If you talk to parents, there is little doubt that what a child eats plays at least a minor role in ADHD symptoms. With the lack of "real" food and the era of synthetic nutrition (foods fortified with synthetic nutrients missing due to modern manufacturing practices) gripping industrialized countries, it is hard to eat better. But it is worth it! You will either pay a little more now for healthier whole foods or a lot later in adverse health conditions. The bottom line is that we can do better to provide cleaner, more nutritious food to all children, but especially those with ADHD.

Common Food Sensitivities in Children with ADHD[259]	
Artificial Food Colorings	Red #40, Red #2, Blue #2, Yellow #5 (Tartrazine), Yellow #6 (Sunset Yellow)
Nonsalicylate Foods	Milk, chocolate, soy, eggs, wheat, corn, legumes
Salicylate Foods	Tomatoes, grapes, oranges

Restore Optimal Levels of Nutrients That May Be Deficient

The human brain depends on a constant supply of glucose, healthy fats, protein (amino acids), and micronutrients (vitamins and minerals) to function optimally. It is so glucose dependent that the brain uses about 20 percent of the body's total supply of glucose for its energy needs.[260] The brain requires the right amino acids and fats to grow new connections (links between regions of the brain) and add myelin to nerves. Amino acids act as precursors (starting materials) to create key neurotransmitters: aspartic acid (aspartate), choline (acetylcholine), glutamic acid (glutamate), phenylalanine (dopamine), tryptophan (serotonin), and tyrosine (norepinephrine). The abundance of these key nutrients available to the brain affects neuronal, cognitive, and mental function, and behavior, memory, and learning.

Glucose

Some tissues in the body can use protein or fat as an energy source, but the brain can only use glucose. The brain's glucose supply comes from carbohydrates consumed by way of glucose metabolism (the process whereby simple sugars from foods are processed and used to produce energy in the form of adenosine triphosphate (ATP). ATP is the energy currency of life—a high-energy molecule that stores the energy required for virtually everything we do. Dietary carbohydrates (whole grains, vegetables—squash, zucchini, honey, and potatoes, to name a few) provide glucose from polysaccharides (ten or more glucose units), oligosaccharides (three to nine glucose units), disaccharides—lactose, sucrose, and maltose (two glucose units), and monosaccharides (one glucose molecule). Glucose not required immediately for energy needs is stored in the body (the liver is an important storage site) as glycogen. When needed, stored glycogen is released and converted to glucose by a process called gluconeogenesis. Other precursors used by the body to form glucose include pyruvate, amino acids, and glycerol. As you can imagine, the brain controls the amount of glucose available to it very tightly and regularly stimulates the release and storage of glucose based on its needs.

Interestingly, studies using positron emission tomography (PET) scans discovered that brain areas that control attention use less glucose in people with ADHD. This phenomenon suggests that these areas of the brain are less active and slower due to lack of energy supply, which may contribute to inattention and other symptoms.[261] Other research suggests that low blood sugar levels may contribute to inattention and impulsivity.[262,263] Some research even discovered that exposure to amphetamines appears to at least partially work by stimulating glucose uptake in the frontal lobes of the brain.[264] Brain activity is highly dependent on glucose availability and utilization, and when less glucose is available, the brain will send distress messages that may increase carbohydrate cravings. The key is to get wholesome carbohydrates with multiple glucose units (complex carbohydrates) to provide the brain the fuel it needs without introducing simple sugars and refined carbohydrates.

Omega-3 Fatty Acids

Omega-3 fatty acids, also called n-3 polyunsaturated fatty acids (PUFAs), are healthy fats that are vital for human health. They are called essential fatty acids (EFAs) because the body can't make them from other fats and requires a steady supply from food. Omega-3s are an integral part of cell membranes, which affects the function of cell receptors in these membranes. They are also used to create hormones that regulate blood clotting, vasodilation, and inflammation. In addition, omega-3s bind to cell receptors to regulate genetic function. Foods high in omega-3s include fish, vegetable oils, nuts, flaxseeds, and leafy vegetables. There are three main types of omega-3s:

- Alpha-linolenic acid (ALA) is the most common omega-3 obtained in most Western diets. It is found in vegetable oils, nuts, flaxseeds, leafy vegetables, and animal fat from grass-fed animals. It is used by the body for energy and converted to EPA and DHA (although this conversion is very limited).
- Eicosapentaenoic acid (EPA) is found in cold-water fatty fish. It serves as a precursor for the production of prostaglandin-3 (which inhibits platelet aggregation), leukotriene-5 eicosanoids (which reduce inflammation), and thromboxane-3 (which promote vasodilation and mildly inhibit platelet aggregation).
- Docosahexaenoic acid (DHA) also comes mainly from fish, with small amounts found in red algae. It is the primary structural component of the brain (cerebral cortex), skin, retina, testicles, and sperm. It is also used to create compounds (resolvins, protectins, and maresins) that reduce inflammation.[265,266] DHA is considered the most important of the omega-3s and the primary omega-3 responsible for the benefits we get after consuming them.

Omega-3s play a vital role in normal growth and development, brain function, and behavior. They encourage positive expression of genes responsible for synaptic function (improving neuronal cellular communication) and plasticity (critical to memory and learning).[267] On the contrary, saturated fats (and refined sugar for that matter) reduce cognitive abilities, negatively affect neuroplasticity (the ability to reorganize pathways in the brain based on experiences, which allow the learning and memorization of new information), and increase neurological dysfunction.[268,269] The balance of omega-3s to saturated fats in the diet of children with ADHD therefore becomes vitally important.

Scientists have observed that deficiencies in EFAs produces symptoms similar to ADHD.[270,271] Studies also demonstrate that deficiencies in omega-3s contributes to learning and behavioral problems connected with ADHD.[272] One study observed that boys aged six to twelve years with low levels of omega-3s experienced a greater frequency of temper tantrums, trouble sleeping, and learning and health problems, according to reports by their parents.[273] Additional research suggests that providing more omega-3s to children with ADHD significantly reduces the number and severity of a wide variety of ADHD symptoms.[274] The evidence is mounting in support of including more omega-3s in the diet to improve both behavior and learning of children with ADHD.[275]

Aim to include more omega-3 fats and less trans (manmade fat that is considered the most harmful to human health) and saturated fats and monitor if your child's ADHD symptoms improve. It is important to note that ALA is converted to DHA or EPA after consumption, but this conversion may not occur effectively.[276,277] This is unfortunate because research suggests that DHA and EPA are more biologically active and beneficial than ALA.[278] The challenge is that EPA and DHA are predominantly found in fish, something a child is not as likely to consume. However, benefits and a better omega-3-to-saturated-fats balance can be achieved through marine oil supplements—more to come about this in the next chapter.[279,280]

This recommendation would also include women who are pregnant because the availability of DHA during pregnancy plays a vital role in the proper development and function of the brain.

Zinc and Iron

Deficiencies or reduced levels of zinc and iron have been observed in some children with ADHD.[281] Both zinc and iron are critical to neurological function. Sufficient iron is necessary to produce neurotransmitters and myelin, and inadequate iron levels cause dysregulation of dopamine levels.[282,283] Abnormal iron levels are associated with negative effects on cognition due to variations in brain structure integrity, particularly white matter and myelin.[284] What the scientists observed was that the amount of iron obtained in the diet as a teenager is strongly associated with brain integrity as an adult. Cognitive and learning difficulties have also been observed in children with low iron levels.[285] The brain must tightly control iron levels within a narrow range to optimize cognition and brain development and reduce the risk of neurodegeneration. Too much or too little iron in the brain can cause cognitive and neurological impairment.

The best way to get iron is through foods rich in it. Iron supplements are generally unnecessary unless a deficiency or low levels are confirmed during a blood test. Some foods rich in iron include red meat, pork, chicken, turkey, fish, beans, spinach, dried fruit, blackstrap molasses, and quinoa.

Zinc's role in shortening the duration of the common cold is well known, but few realize its magnitude in brain function. The highest amounts of zinc are found in the brain, particularly the hippocampus. Zinc is important for normal brain function, neuronal communication, neurotransmitter production, and the prevention of neurological diseases.[286,287] Zinc helps regulate communication between neurons and the hippocampus, which helps improve memory and learning abilities.[288] In addition, it binds to the dopamine transporter, which slows it down and keeps dopamine active in the synapse for a longer period of time.

This action is similar to stimulant medications used to treat ADHD and increases dopamine's action on mood, attention, memory, learning, and movement.

Another reason zinc may play a role in ADHD is its action as a cofactor to the enzyme delta-6-desaturate—an enzyme crucial to fatty acid metabolism (think back to our EFA discussion above).[289,290] If inadequate zinc is present, this enzyme may not be active to break down fats and assimilate these key fatty acids into cells and tissues that rely on them for proper function. Low zinc levels in children have been linked to hyperactivity, aggression, impaired learning, boredom, and mental retardation.[291,292] Middle Eastern countries where zinc deficiency is more common have reported a high number of children with ADHD have very low zinc levels.[293] Boosting zinc in the diet is a viable option if a known zinc deficiency exists.

The importance of zinc to the activity of hundreds of enzymes and human health in general make it even more important to get an adequate supply of zinc from the food we eat. Few foods provide high amounts of zinc, which requires incorporating a number of foods with good levels of zinc into the diet. In addition, plant sources also contain phytic acid, which binds to zinc and decreases its bioavailability, making vegetarians more vulnerable to deficiencies. Foods that are a good source of zinc include beef, lamb, sesame seeds, pumpkin seeds, lentils, garbanzo beans, cashews, turkey, and quinoa.

Magnesium

Magnesium serves as a cofactor for at least three hundred enzymatic reactions and is crucial for fatty acid production. It plays a vital role in protecting brain structure and function throughout aging, and it is a key nutrient for optimal nervous system function. Magnesium is involved in synaptic plasticity (the ability of synapses to strengthen or weaken in response to neurotransmitter levels in a synapse) and density (accumulation of material on the postsynaptic membrane).[294,295,296] Synaptic plasticity and density encourages rapid retrieval and processing of information, which enhances learning and memory. Low magnesium levels have been reported in children with ADHD.[297,298] Preliminary evidence suggests that restoring magnesium levels to optimum ranges may reduce hyperactivity, impulsivity, and inattention. Given that a preliminary study found that 72 percent of children are magnesium-deficient, and increasing these levels improved ADHD symptoms,[299] magnesium levels should be regularly checked in individuals with ADHD.

Magnesium is a key mineral found in a variety of foods. Despite its wide availability in foods, the typical American diet frequently fails to meet the body's needs for this important nutrient. Foods that have good levels of magnesium include pumpkin seeds, spinach, Swiss chard, sesame seeds, quinoa, black beans, cashews, sunflower seeds, avocado, and almonds. You may have noticed that some of the same foods are repeated for the various nutrients (quinoa, seeds, beans), suggesting they may be key foods for the person with ADHD.

Vitamin D

Vitamin D is quickly being recognized as one of the most important nutrients to human health. Remarkably higher blood levels of vitamin D significantly alters the activity of 291 genes and more than 160 biological pathways linked to cancer, cardiovascular disease, and autoimmune disorders.[300] It also controls up to 5 percent of the human genome (the complete set of genetic material that makes up humans).[301] Vitamin D receptors are widespread in brain tissue, and it serves to guide neurons to specific regions of the brain that shape its structure and function, implying it plays a significant role in cognitive function.[302] Interestingly, vitamin D receptors, or the enzymes needed to convert vitamin D to its active form, are concentrated in areas of the brain that may be abnormal in children with ADHD (prefrontal cortex, hippocampus, cingulated gyrus, and substantia nigra).[303,304] Vitamin D is also involved in the differentiation (how generic cells become specialized cells that perform a specific function in humans) of developing brain cells. Children with behavioral disorders like ADHD tend to have lower levels of vitamin D.[305] Given the far-reaching benefits to human health of vitamin D, it would be unwise to exclude this nutrient from your daily diet.

Vitamin D interacts with cell receptors throughout the body, which means it is better classified as a hormone than a vitamin (hormone D, not vitamin D). Unfortunately, it is found only in small amounts in foods, making it difficult to get an adequate— let alone an optimal—supply of this critically important nutrient. Foods highest in vitamin D include cod liver oil, oily fish (salmon, swordfish, white fish, mackerel, trout, and tuna), mushrooms (Maitake, Portobello), pork, and eggs. A number of foods are also fortified with vitamin D (cereal, dairy products, dairy substitutes, and juice), but these usually contain the synthetic and less bioavailable form of vitamin D, vitamin D2.

Changing your child's diet to include these nutrients more frequently may profoundly influence his or her ADHD symptoms alone, but greater benefits are more likely when combined with other natural therapies. In addition, if deficiency exists, it is vital to restore optimal levels of key nutrients to ensure optimal brain function. It is not easy to make changes in a child's diet—especially drastic ones—but it will be worth it if it leads to noticeable improvements. At the very least, you will be providing your child with more nutritious meals that could lead to better health as an adult.

Rebuild Gut Health and Restore Intestinal Balance

Proper digestion and absorption of nutrients is critical to overall health. Without optimum digestion, many nutrients will pass through the digestive tract unabsorbed or, worse, could remain as undigested residue that damages the mucosal membrane and triggers an immune cascade that wreaks havoc in the body. This type of environment is less than ideal for health to thrive and opens the door for diseases and adverse conditions to occur, including neurological disorders.

Intestinal permeability is the ability of the intestines to maintain tight junctions and allow beneficial substances to exit through the intestinal wall into the bloodstream while keeping harmful substances inside the intestines for elimination. In other words, intestinal permeability serves as the gatekeeper from your intestines to the bloodstream. It rejects substances that may do harm by tightly closing the entrance door, and opens the door just enough for beneficial substances to enter. This process protects humans from invasion by harmful organisms and toxins and allows the absorption of essential oil fluids and nutrients. This process must be tightly regulated for optimum human health.

Billions of bacteria—both good and bad—line the mucosal surface of the digestive tract and the largest immune system of the body (up to 80 percent of the immune system lies within the gut). Both types of bacteria are constantly waging a war for more real estate in your intestines. The microbiome balance that results from this war significantly influences intestinal permeability. When the bad guys gain ground, intestinal permeability increases allowing the release of pathogens, toxins, and allergens into the bloodstream.[306,307,308] On the other hand, when the good guys maintain a proper balance and a diversity of organisms is present, the integrity of this barrier to harmful substances is preserved.[309,310,311] We have two choices in our diet, support the good guys with fermented foods or let the bad guys run amuck.

The more we learn about probiotics (live bacteria and yeasts that inhabit the skin, mouth, sexual organs, and, especially, the intestines that are beneficial to health) and their influence on overall well-being, the clearer it becomes that probiotics are one of the most important dietary supplements for people of all ages. This is also true with brain health as emerging research reveals the role of probiotics in brain health and function.[312,313,314,315] An increased understanding of gut bacteria, part of the human microbiome, suggests that the sooner a healthy microbiome is established—often by introducing healthy bacteria during infancy—the better a child's health will be.[316,317,318,319,320] A mounting body of evidence even suggests that early colonization of the gut environment with probiotics (called microbial programming) may reduce the risk of diseases later in life.[321,322,323] The simple and inexpensive practice of providing probiotics throughout life—from infants to the elderly—can have a long-lasting positive influence on overall well-being.

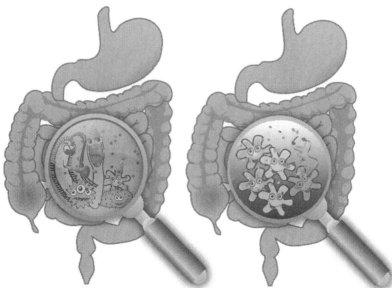

Who is winning the battle in your gut? The balance between healthy to harmful bacteria can significantly influence your overall well-being and risk for disease.

Exposures to and interactions with microbial communities during the course of human history have influenced virtually all aspects of human health, including physiology, metabolism, and behavior. This evolution of the gut microbiome from that of our hunter-gatherer ancestors to modern day has largely been influenced by diet and the introduction of drugs into the gut.[324] Accelerated scientific investigations have revealed how these microscopic organisms interface with the immune, central nervous, enteric nervous, musculoskeletal, and cardiovascular systems.[325,326,327,328] Indeed, researchers now recognize the importance of early colonization of the gut for optimum immune system function.[329,330] Based on these advances, probiotic therapy has been recommended for the treatment and prevention of a host of disorders from allergies to irritable bowel syndrome, and autoimmune diseases to behavioral disorders.[331]

The lining of your gastrointestinal tract is the largest surface area that interacts with your external environment.[332] Billions of biological sensors (nerve cells, endocrine cells, and immune cells) line the intestinal tract to identify the constituents of the intestinal environment. All of these biological sensors are profoundly influenced by the gut microbiome and the balance of probiotics to harmful organisms residing in the digestive tract. Based on what these cells detect, they send signals throughout the body that influence the function of tissues and organs, all of which leads to remarkable benefits body-wide—especially in relation to metabolism, immunity, and inflammation.

Symbiosis—which translates to "living in harmony"—occurs when a healthy balance and diversity of microbes is present. Some experts consider the optimal ratio of good to bad bacteria in the digestive tract to be 85 percent good and 15 percent bad. Dysbiosis is the medical term for imbalanced or less diverse microbiota in the gut. It is when the "bad guys" take over the digestive tract or one particular strain is dominating it. Normally the balance of good to harmful bacteria constantly living in the digestive tract keep each other in check so that dysbiosis doesn't occur. However, typically harmless bacteria living in the digestive tract can trigger mild to serious health issues, including those of psychological origin when dysbiosis is present.[333]

An investigation published by Finnish researchers in 2015 brought gut microbiome health to the forefront of the ADHD discussion. During the study seventy-five infants were randomized to one of two groups. Group one received the probiotic Lactobacillus rhamnosus for the first six months of life, while the second group received a placebo. The children were followed over the course of thirteen years. At the study's conclusion just over 17 percent of the children in the placebo group were diagnosed with ADHD or Asperger's syndrome (an autism spectrum disorder).[334] Astonishingly, not a single child who received the probiotic supplement as an infant was diagnosed with either ADHD or Asperger's syndrome. Evidence from this study is very compelling and quite convincing that a healthy gut microbiome is one of the most fundamental initiators of health.

While this research merits further study with a larger sample size, it demonstrates the profound influence a symbiotic microbiome can have on overall health. It also suggests that introducing a single species of probiotic into the gut microbiome during infancy can be enormously beneficial. The question now becomes—What benefits could be achieved with a multispecies probiotic including several clinically proven strains? Again, it is such a simple and inexpensive thing to administer to infants with very little, if any risk, and huge potential. Why are we not mandating probiotics for infants during the first several months of life?

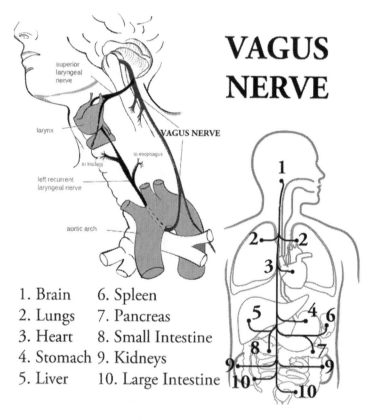

1. Brain
2. Lungs
3. Heart
4. Stomach
5. Liver
6. Spleen
7. Pancreas
8. Small Intestine
9. Kidneys
10. Large Intestine

The gut-brain axis is a two-way communication system between the enteric nervous system (found in the gastrointestinal tract and often referred to as the "second brain") and the central nervous system. The state of the gut microbiome significantly influences this communication and healthy brain function. Signals are transmitted via the vagus nerve, which extends from the brainstem to the abdomen by way of multiple organs (i.e., the heart, esophagus, and lungs). It is actually two cranial nerves (left and right) that regulate a variety of body functions, such as heartbeat, respiratory muscle movement, and the amounts of digestive chemicals used to process food. Malfunction of the vagus nerve can lead to a variety of problems in several body systems.

Interestingly, up to 90 percent of signaling along the vagus nerve is from the gastrointestinal tract to the brain, suggesting a great deal of autonomy for the enteric nervous system. In essence, the vagus nerve acts as a switchboard for the autonomic nervous system and its impairment can lead to a number of health challenges. In reality, some neurological disorders actually begin in the gut and spread upward to the brain via the vagus nerve.[335,336] The vagus nerve and the enteric nervous system are responsible for our gut instinct and butterflies in the stomach. As a matter of fact, these feelings are responses to nerve signals.

One of the most effective ways to improve microbiome balance is to consume fermented foods like yogurt (cultured coconut milk yogurt is a good option to avoid processed dairy), kefir, sauerkraut, pickles, fermented vegetables (carrots, squash, etc.), kimchi, and kvass. Just be careful with some products (like standard yogurt) that are loaded with sugar. Your average probiotic supplement contains from two to thirty billion live colony-forming units (CFUs) of probiotics. Compare this to fermented vegetables that can have up to ten trillion CFUs, and clearly the right fermented foods give you more bang for your buck.

CFUs in Some Fermented Foods	
Yogurt (4 oz.)	90 to 500 billion[337]
Sauerkraut (1 cup)	1.42 billion[338]
Kefir (4 oz.)	118 billion[339,340]

Conclusion

The bottom line is that optimizing digestion should be one of the first therapies considered by both parents and physicians who work with a child with ADHD. Greater efforts should be made to identify potential trigger foods, provide well-balanced meals with adequate high-quality protein, reduce empty calories, optimize nutrient levels, rebuild gut health, and restore intestinal balance. The far-reaching benefits of eating better can't be overstated. Your great efforts may be rewarded with a more balanced child and reduced ADHD symptoms.

5

EVIDENCE-BASED ALTERNATIVES FOR ADHD—
SUPPLEMENTS AND ESSENTIAL OILS

The majority of therapies offered for ADHD from Western medicine focus on balancing chemicals in the brain. Fortunately, Mother Nature has provided for natural options that can also influence the levels of these chemicals available to the brain and therefore reduce ADHD symptoms. One of the challenges with natural alternatives for ADHD is that there are so many opinions as to what will help, and these opinions are often just that— opinions that don't have a lot of support in science. Certainly, positive testimonials from parents, teachers, and clinicians should be considered, but for the purpose of this chapter, we will focus on evidence-based alternatives.

Essential Fatty Acids (DHA, EPA, and Gamma Linolenic Acid)

We have previously established the importance of healthy fats in the chapter on nutrition. Marine animals consume EFA-rich algae and then concentrate DHA and EPA in their tissues. Because of the poor conversion from ALA (plant-based EFAs) to DHA in humans, it is ideal that the body receive DHA directly. As stated earlier, a significant challenge with getting EFAs by way of nutrition is the fact that many children do not like the taste of fish. If this is the case with your child, then a high-quality fish oil supplement may be an option.

The human brain undergoes its most rapid and complex growth during the last trimester of pregnancy and during the first two years of life. Over the course of the last trimester the brain grows approximately 260 percent and grows an additional 193 percent through age two (roughly 175 percent in year one and 18 percent in year two). During this time, the brain requires a constant flow of essential nutrients, especially DHA, for optimal neurological development.[341,342] From the age of two to adulthood the brain only grows an additional 21 percent, with most brain growth completed by age five or six. In addition, EFAs are critical to the production of neurotransmitters. So you have a short time period to fuel the brain with the right nutrients to grow and develop optimally.

Your brain is predominantly fat—approximately 60 percent of the brain is made of fat.[343] It is estimated that 30 percent of your total brain fat is DHA, which is predominantly located in the forebrain (the front of the brain, including the cerebral hemispheres, thalamus, and hypothalamus and the part of the brain most used for sustained attention). The forebrain rapidly accumulates DHA during the first two years of life, but not other fats.[344] This means that DHA is likely the most important fat for developing children's brains.

Researchers have evaluated the effect of fatty acid availability during pregnancy and the resulting behavioral outcomes as a child. German researchers completed an eleven-year study that assessed fatty acid levels present in the umbilical cord blood at birth. Data on children's behavior was collected at age ten among the 416 children included in the study. Remarkably, what the researchers found was that a 1 percent increase in DHA in cord blood decreased total behavioral and emotional difficulties significantly.[345] This added evidence to previous research that found mothers who supplemented with EPA and DHA had children with higher mental processing scores, psychomotor development (the progressive attainment of mental and muscular activity by a child; i.e. learning to crawl, walk, and talk), eye-hand coordination, and stereoacuity (the ability to detect the depth or distance of an object) at age four.[346,347] It can't be stressed enough how important getting optimal levels of DHA and EPA is during pregnancy, especially considering their extensive safety record.

Developing babies require their DHA supply from their mothers. The amount of DHA in a mother's breast milk is highly variable depending on the mother's diet.[348,349] If the mother eats a diet high in fish and seafood, she will have a greater supply of DHA for her developing baby during pregnancy and lactation. If her diet lacks marine foods, she should take a fish oil supplement to provide the nutrients necessary for optimum neurological development. Most infant formulas are also fortified with DHA for those mothers who choose not to breastfeed. Some experts recommend that pregnant women supplement with omega-3s (1,000 mg of DHA daily) and a neuroprotective antioxidant (600 mg of n-acetyl cysteine, twice daily) to prevent ADHD, autism spectrum, and cerebral palsy.[350] The bottom line is that your baby needs optimum levels of DHA during these critical brain growth periods to have the most positive cognitive outcomes later in life.

According to some experts, boys require three times more fatty acids than girls do.[351] This is interesting since boys tend to be diagnosed with ADHD disproportionately compared to girls. A hypothesis is that this phenomenon may be due to higher levels of estrogen in women, which helps transport fatty acids to the brain and other tissues; whereas testosterone (the primary male sex hormone) is not a fatty acid carrier. Another factor that affects all children, but may add to the already present deficit in boys, is the fact that modern diets are deficient in healthy fats. Both of these reasons contribute to a perfect storm for DHA brain starvation to occur in boys. Fortunately, DHA supplementation (1,200 mg per day) has been shown to improve cortical function—an area of the brain associated with sustained attention over time (vigilance).[352]

DHA is vital for the ongoing structure and function of the adult brain as well. DHA is vital to cell membrane fluidity (the degree of rigidity of the lipid bilayer that surrounds cells), which influences cell permeability, cellular function, and cell signaling. In other words, higher concentrations of DHA improves communication between brain cells. DHA's unique structural properties and influence on cell membrane function is credited for the expansion of gray matter levels in the cerebral cortex over the course of human history.[353,354] Indeed, modern science has discovered that people with higher concentrations of

DHA in the brain have greater total brain volume and improved memory and executive function.[355,356] This is important because those suffering with ADHD typically have less gray matter in their brain.

Low levels of DHA are associated with ADHD symptoms, antisocial traits, and a poorer quality of life.[357,358] Conversely, optimizing DHA levels can lead to reduced ADHD symptoms and improved quality of life. DHA, alone or in combination with gamma-linoleic acid (GLA; found in borage oil and evening primrose oil) has been shown to improve ADHD symptoms such as poor attention and behavior.[359,360] Boys with and without ADHD who received 650 mg each of DHA and EPA daily were rated as more attentive by their parents.[361] Another study found that oppositional behavior, hyperactivity, inattention, and cognitive problems were reduced with an EPA/DHA supplement.[362] When 635 mg of EPA and 195 mg of DHA were given daily to 103 children aged six to twelve years for eight weeks, they experienced reduced ADHD symptoms, inflammation, and oxidative stress.[363] Research is mixed with DHA and EPA in the reduction of ADHD symptoms, but the negative studies have generally used isolated DHA and less than 515 mg of DHA per day in children aged six to twelve, suggesting DHA and EPA should be taken toghether and higher intakes may be necessary to realize benefits.[364,365] Highlighted by the data in these studies is the fact that it takes high levels of DHA and EPA to experience clinical benefits. Molecularly distilled fish oils naturally concentrate the DHA and EPA to higher levels.

Some research suggests that supplementing with DHA and EPA may be of particular importance among children with ADHD who also experience learning difficulties. Australian researchers gave children (seven to twelve years of age) 1373 mg EPA and 1140 mg of DHA daily for four months. After four months, the researchers found that a specific subset of children with learning difficulties and ADHD experienced improved reading, spelling, and ability to divide attention, as well as reduced hyperactivity, restlessness, and overall ADHD symptoms.[366] Interestingly, the other children with ADHD did not experience significant improvements compared to the control group.

Some emerging research suggests that triglyceride (TG) forms of fish oil may be the most beneficial, although most clinical studies utilize the ethyl ester (EE) type.[367] Unrefined fish oil in its natural state contains triglycerides with DHA and EPA that are attached to glycerol. When fish oil is molecularly distilled to remove harmful substances (heavy metals, dioxins, PCBs, and other toxins present in fish), the glycerol molecule is also removed, which converts the fish oil to the EE type. Some manufacturers add the glycerol molecule back into the fish oil after processing, which returns it to a TG form. This may increase both the bioavailability and the effectiveness of your fish oil supplements. Based on the available research the following are suggested doses of EPA and DHA (from marine oils) to reduce the risk of ADHD during pregnancy and lactation and to manage symptoms:

- Pregnancy and lactation: 1,000–1,500 mg DHA and 500–750 mg EPA daily
- Age two to four: 500–750 mg DHA and 250–350 mg EPA
- Age four to eight: 750–1,000 mg DHA and 250–500 mg EPA
- Age nine to seventeen: 1,250–1,500 mg DHA and 750–1,000 mg EPA
- 18+: Experts suggest that healthy adults obtain 650 mg each of DHA\EPA daily,[368] those with ADHD may require higher levels such as 1,500–2,000 mg DHA and 1,000–1,250 mg EPA

Gamma linolenic acid (GLA) is an omega-6 fatty acid—another type of polyunsaturated fatty acid—primarily found in vegetable oils. Along with omega-3s, omega-6 fatty acids play an essential role in brain function. The majority of vegetable oils provide the omega-6 fatty acid linoleic acid (LA), which the body converts to GLA and arachidonic acid (AA). The modern Westernized diet consists of far too many omega-6 fatty acids in comparison to omega-3s—on average fourteen to twenty-five times more. The problem with this out of balance ratio is that some omega-6 fatty acids—both LA and AA—increase inflammation. GLA is an exception to this rule and actually decreases inflammation because the body converts it to a substance called DGLA (dihomo gamma linolenic acid).[369,370] In order to convert GLA to DGLA the body must have sufficient levels of key nutrients like magnesium, zinc, and vitamins C, B3, and B6. While GLA does decrease inflammation, it is not as potent an anti-inflammatory as omega-3s.

Scientific research surrounding the use of GLA for ADHD is mixed. One shortcoming of many studies with GLA and ADHD is that they administer both LA (inflammatory) with the GLA. One study with thirty-one children administered 2,160 mg of LA and 270 mg of GLA, or a placebo, for four weeks. After four weeks of supplementation the parents and teachers reported improved attention and less hyperactivity.[371] Another study that was longer in duration (twelve weeks) gave higher doses (2,800 mg LA and 320 mg GLA) daily. The study authors did not observe any significant benefits after twelve weeks.[372] A third study administered both omega-3s (558 EPA mg and 174 mg DHA daily) and GLA (60 mg daily) to seventy-five children for six months. What the researchers found was that nearly half of the children experienced reduced ADHD symptoms at the end of the six-month study.[373] Based on the available research, DHA and EPA should be the first line of defense when it comes to fatty acid supplementation, while GLA could be considered if no positive response occurs with DHA and EPA.

Vitamin D

Vitamin D is frequently combined with fish oil in clinical trials. A great number of the world population have less than optimal levels of vitamin D today. Vitamin D is required to activate an enzyme (tryptophan hydroxylase 2) that triggers the production of serotonin. Insufficient levels of vitamin D during pregnancy and early childhood may cause psychological problems and unfavorable effects on brain development, structure, and function.[374,375] In addition, both DHA and EPA are influential in the release and function of serotonin in the brain. Another nutrient that promotes balance of key neurotransmitters, EPA reduces prostaglandins to increase serotonin release, whereas DHA increases cell membrane fluidity in neurons to increase the brains response to serotonin. Scientists now hypothesize that deficiencies in vitamin D and omega-3s, along with genetic factors, may lead to neurological disorders like ADHD and impulsive behavior.[376]

Vitamin D deficiency is common in people with ADHD;[377,378] however, vitamin D deficiency is common among global populations generally. Studies estimate that the prevalence of vitamin D deficiency is almost 42 percent among the total population of the United States, with higher rates seen among African-Americans (82.1%) and Hispanics (69.2%).[379] Darker colored skin reduces the synthesis of vitamin D from sun exposure by as much as 99 percent,[380,381] which may at least partially account for greater deficiencies among African-Americans and Hispanics. World populations don't fare much better when it comes to vitamin D deficiency. It is estimated that upwards of 30 to 50 percent of children and adults worldwide are at risk of vitamin D deficiency.[382,383,384,385,386,387] Because of this, it is more difficult to correlate vitamin D status as a causal factor in ADHD, but it is well-known that it is a vital nutrient involved in brain function.

One thing for certain is that vitamin D plays a role in boosting levels of the antioxidant glutathione in the brain by regulating the enzyme gamma-glutamyl transpeptidase (GGT).[388,389,390] GGT helps recycle glutathione, which makes more of it available to the body. Glutathione can quickly be depleted in the brain if it is not recycled for reuse efficiently. And glutathione is necessary to recycle other antioxidants. Think of glutathione as the final processer of free radicals. Other antioxidants like vitamins C and E assault the free radical first and then hand it off to glutathione to obliterate. In turn, glutathione replenishes vitamins C and E so they can go attack other free radicals.

Glutathione is the master detoxifier, but poor diet, toxins, excess stress, aging, infections, and pollution all deplete glutathione levels in the body. Insufficient glutathione levels leave you more susceptible to cellular damage and destruction caused by oxidative stress, infections, and cancer. Your liver is the primary organ of detoxification and relies on glutathione to do its job. Glutathione is also a key antioxidant involved in brain detoxification. Through chelation (bonding to and excreting another substance), glutathione helps rid the brain of heavy metals, protects neurons, and improves neuronal communication that is vital to cognition.[391,392,393,394,395] It is also noteworthy that deficits in antioxidants and decreased antioxidant activity may aggravate ADHD symptoms.[396] When you consider this role of vitamin D, it may indirectly influence ADHD symptoms.

Vitamin D is another vitamin that is important to get optimal levels of during pregnancy. Higher vitamin D levels among mothers is associated with a lower risk of ADHD-like symptoms among their children.[397] For every 10 ng/ml increase in vitamin D levels in expectant mothers, their children realize an 11 percent decreased risk of ADHD-like symptoms. Pregnant women should work with their health professional to determine current their vitamin D status and the need for a supplement to augment vitamin D levels.

It is a good practice for children to take a vitamin D supplement for general health purposes. Even Western physicians recognize and encourage this practice. The American Academy of Pediatrics recommends infants receive 400 IU of vitamin D daily beginning soon after birth and up until they are weaned from nursing and taking vitamin D-fortified milk. However, if vitamin D deficiency or insufficiency exists, it is even more important to supplement with this very important nutrient. Evidence strongly suggests that children and adolescents need 2,000 IU of vitamin D daily to achieve desirable levels.[398,399] Again, current levels should be determined by a health professional to customize a proper dose to achieve optimum levels (targeting 50 nmol/L).

Zinc and Iron

Enzymes are present in every living cell. They serve to power body functions by accelerating chemical reactions. An amazing number of chemical reactions is possible in the body, each of which is regulated by enzymes. Enzymes manufacture products of these chemical reactions quickly and efficiently by combining with other substances (called a substrate). However, enzymes require cofactors (like minerals) to work. There are eighteen known cofactors: calcium, chlorine, chromium, cobalt, copper, fluorine, iodide, iron, magnesium, manganese, molybdenum, phosphorus, potassium, selenium, sodium, sulfur, vanadium, and zinc. Some cofactors can work interchangeably, which is your body's built-in survival mechanism when one cofactor is not available because of an unbalanced diet. A better plan is to ensure optimal levels of cofactors through diet and supplementation.

Mineral deficiencies are commonly reported in children with ADHD, particularly zinc and iron.[400,401,402,403,404] Iron is a cofactor for brain structure and function, growth and development in children, essential to hemoglobin production, involved in immune system defenses, and vital for cell survival. Zinc is a cofactor for over one hundred enzymes, including those involved in dopamine transport, brain structure and function, muscle contractions, prostate health, insulin formation, and the synthesis of DNA. If insufficient levels of either iron or zinc are available in the body, hundreds of enzymes may not perform chemical reactions that are vital to life.

Persons with insufficiencies or deficiencies of minerals are more likely to have positive results when supplementing with them. Curiously, supplementing with zinc alongside stimulant medications has been shown to increase the effectiveness of the drugs and reduce the required dose by up to 37 percent.[405] Similar findings have been observed with iron supplements.[406] This suggests that mineral cofactors may improve medication responses or reduce medication or both requirements—a positive finding that could reduce the number and severity of side effects to medications.

Serum-zinc levels in children directly correlate with parent- and teacher-rated inattention in children with ADHD.[407] When a child has lower serum-zinc levels his parents and teachers are more inclined to rate him as more symptomatic. Guatemalan researchers tested the effect of supplementing children with ADHD with 10 mg of zinc five days per week for six months. The scientists observed little change in ADHD symptoms, but anxiety and depression symptoms were reduced as zinc concentrations increased in the blood.[408] While no direct effect of zinc was observed, it is positive that emotional symptoms were alleviated by the zinc supplement. Emotional disorders can trigger behavioral disorders, so greater mood balance may impact ADHD-symptoms.

Chilean researchers conducted a small pilot study that administered 0.3 mg/kg daily of zinc along with stimulant medications. After six weeks, a small improvement in ADHD symptoms was observed in the group receiving zinc and medications.[409] Similar findings were observed in an Iranian study that administered 1 mg/kg of zinc daily with stimulant medications.[410] Another study that included 218 Turkish students demonstrated that 15 mg of elemental zinc syrup daily reduced inattentiveness, hyperactivity, and oppositional behavior.[411] Significant positive results were obtained when high doses of zinc (105mg/day) were administered without medication for twelve weeks.[412] Researchers concluded that this high dose of zinc significantly reduced hyperactivity, impulsivity, and impaired socialization, but did not have an effect on inattentive symptoms. Based on this result, it seems that zinc works best on the hyperactive-impulsive subtype of ADHD. These results may be at least partially explained by the ability of zinc to influence GABA receptors, which slows overall brain activity. Zinc dosage should be determined by a physician, because therapeutic doses will likely exceed the upper limits established for zinc (ranging from 7 to 34 mg for children aged two to eighteen).

Evidence suggests that insufficient iron levels are associated with increased hyperactivity symptoms, as reported by parents and teachers.[413,414,415] This is likely due to the disruption of dopamine signaling. Low levels of iron have also been linked to sleep problems in children with ADHD.[416] If your child with ADHD has trouble sleeping, low iron levels should be ruled out as a causal factor. Restless legs syndrome has also been reported in children with iron deficiency and ADHD.[417,418] Children with ADHD and restless legs syndrome should have low iron levels ruled out as a cause. Interestingly, children with the inattentive subtype of ADHD are more likely to have iron deficiency. This helps explain the findings of a Spanish study. Spanish scientists found that iron supplementation was successful or partially effective in 89 percent of children with inattentive ADHD but only partially effective in 13 percent of children with noninattentive subtypes of ADHD.[419]

A small French study investigated the benefits of iron supplementation in children with ADHD. Children aged five to eight received 80 mg of ferrous sulfate daily for twelve weeks. After twelve weeks, the study authors noted that the supplement "was well tolerated" and had "effectiveness comparable to stimulants." When 5 mg/kg of iron sulfate was administered to children in another study, parents reported decreased ADHD symptoms.[420] If iron insufficiency or deficiency exists, or your child has the inattentive subtype of ADHD, trouble sleeping, or experiences restless leg syndrome, it is worth evaluating iron levels to rule it out as a trigger or cause.

Iron sulfate is most commonly used in studies, with doses ranging from 5 mg/kg per day and 80 mg per day. Ferrous succinate and ferrous fumarate or chelated iron are also good iron supplement options. Upper limits for children range from 40 to 45 mg, and therefore exceeding this limit should only be done under the care of a physician.

Magnesium

As was discussed in the previous chapter, magnesium plays a crucial role in fostering communication between various regions of the brain. Synapses are the connections that allow one neuron to communicate with the next. They have the ability to adapt— by changing their shape or function—the intensity of their signals (communication) in response to their activity level. Magnesium is essential to the ability of synapses to adapt. Magnesium reshapes synapses leading to enhanced learning abilities, improved short-term and long-term memory, improved working memory (high-speed memory responsible for temporarily storing and managing information necessary to perform tasks, such as comprehension, learning, and reasoning), and enhanced quality of sleep.[421]

One challenge with magnesium supplements is the great difficulty in increasing magnesium levels in the brain, even when administered intravenously.[422,423] Massachusetts Institute of Technology (MIT) researchers appear to have found a way to overcome this obstacle. They formulated a special form of magnesium called magnesium-L-threonate (MgT) that can be taken orally to maximize magnesium levels in the brain.[424,425] Remarkably, MgT also efficiently transfers to the central nervous system (CNS) and to the spinal fluid. In addition, it enhances the production of neural stem cells—cells used to create new brain cells like neurons, astrocytes, and oligodendrocytes.[426,427,428] Neural stem cells hold great promise in brain repair after injury or disease, so this finding is particularly exciting. This infusion of magnesium into the CNS by MgT profoundly influences neurological function, improves learning, and enhances short- and long-term memory (15 percent and 54 percent respectively, compared to magnesium citrate).[429]

Low magnesium levels are consistently observed in studies among people with ADHD.[430,431,432] Preliminary evidence suggests that magnesium supplements may be beneficial in relieving ADHD symptoms in some children. Small, usually uncontrolled, studies show that magnesium and vitamin B6 supplementation results in improvements in behavior, increased attention, and reduced aggression, hyperactivity, anxiety, and abnormal involuntary facial movements (synkinesis).[433,434] However, the evidence is preliminary, definitely requires further larger and controlled studies, and is far from convincing currently. Interestingly, stimulant medications increase magnesium levels in the blood.[435] Again, if a known deficiency exists, supplementation may be an option.

Typical doses of magnesium supplements are 6 mg/kg of body weight daily combined with 0.6 mg/kg of vitamin B6 in children aged seven to twelve.[436] For example, a child who weighs sixty pounds (27.3 kg) would take 164 mg of magnesium and 16 mg of B6 daily. The exception is MgT because it contains less elemental magnesium per dose compared to other forms (1,000 mg of MgT provides 72 mg of elemental magnesium). Based on the animal study, the adult dose for MgT would be 1,000 mg twice daily. For children, this would roughly equate to 28 mg/kg per day. One caution is that magnesium toxicity is possible at doses of 10 mg/kg/day or in excessive doses, so magnesium supplements should be limited to the tolerable upper Intake Levels (ULs) established by the Institutes of Medicine.[437,438,439]

MAGNESIUM & VITAMIN B6 Tolerable Upper Intake Levels[440,441]		
Age	*Magnesium*	*Vitamin B6*
1–3 years	65 mg	30 mg
4–8 years	110 mg	40 mg
9–13 years	350 mg	60 mg
14–18 years	350 mg	80 mg
19+ years	350 mg	100 mg

MAGNESIUM Daily Doses		
Weight	*Magnesium citrate**	*MgT**
20–31 lbs.	Magnesium: ≤ 65 mg B6: 5–8 mg	254–395 mg
32–57 lbs.	Magnesium: 87–110 mg B6: 9–16 mg	407–725 mg
58–100 lbs.	Magnesium: 158–272 mg B6: 16–27 mg	738–1,272
101–153 lbs.	Magnesium: 275–350 mg B6: 28–42 mg	1,285–1,947 mg
154+ lbs.	Magnesium: ≤ 350 mg B6: 43–100 mg	2,000 mg

* Note: Magnesium citrate levels are adapted to ensure the UL is not exceeded. MgT levels are adapted to ensure the UL for elemental magnesium and the manufacturer's recommendations are not exceeded.

French Maritime Pine Bark Extract, Pycnogenol

French maritime pine bark has been used for centuries for a variety of medicinal purposes. Today, a natural plant extract from the bark standardized to 65 to 75 percent procyanidins, called Pycnogenol, is more commonly used for therapeutic purposes. French maritime pine bark is a potent antioxidant and contains a unique combination of procyanidins, bioflavonoids, and phenolic acids that offer extensive benefits to the cardiovascular, integumentary, and circulatory systems. Much of its benefits is derived from its ability to increase nitric oxide production (which increases blood flow), regulate blood glucose levels, and reduce inflammation. This is important for overall health, as scientists now widely recognize that maintaining normal inflammation and blood sugar levels is a major key to reducing the risk of several of today's most common diseases.

Scientists hypothesize that Pycnogenol may improve blood flow to and antioxidant status in the brain and therefore aid memory and brain function. Italian researchers conducted a study with fifty-three university students aged eighteen to twenty-seven to determine Pycnogenol's effects on brain function. Students were randomly assigned to receive 100 mg of Pycnogenol or a placebo for eight weeks. After eight weeks the study results demonstrated that the Pycnogenol group experienced improvements in attention, mood, and memory, and reduced anxiety.[442] The study results were later confirmed in a subsequent experiment with sixty middle-aged adults (aged thirty-five to fifty-five), demonstrating that Pycnogenol improves executive function, sustained attention, mood, and overall mental performance and cognitive function.[443] Both of these studies showed improvement in already healthy people and provide promising results for people who want to improve mental acuity.

Italian scientists investigated the benefits of Pycnogenol among forty-four elderly persons (age fifty-five to seventy years) in good health but with high levels of oxidative stress. Oxidative stress is a condition where an imbalance in antioxidants to free radicals exists. Impaired brain cell function may occur when oxidative stress is present, and if left unchecked, it may contribute to the development of neurological disorders.[444] Participants in the Italian study were randomly assigned to two groups. One group took 100 mg of Pycnogenol daily and implemented lifestyle changes (sleep at least eight hours, go to bed no later than 10:30, eat regular meals at defined hours, exercise at least twenty minutes daily, and reduce caffeine, salt, sugar, and alcohol intake), whereas the control group only implemented the lifestyle changes. After twelve months, those who took Pycnogenol increased decision-making abilities 71%, memory 37.3%, and attention span 41.2%, while simultaneously reducing oxidative stress by 28%.[445] Conversely, the control group experienced declines in decision-making abilities (5%) and memory (9.8%), a statistically insignificant 1.9% increase in attention span, and no change in oxidative stress levels (they still had high oxidative stress at the end of the study). The study findings are remarkable and demonstrate that Pycnogenol can profoundly influence oxidative stress status and improve cognitive functions.

Pycnogenol has also been investigated in children with ADHD.[446] Sixty-one children were given 1 mg/kg of body weight per day for four weeks as part of a randomized, placebo-controlled, double-blind study. The children were monitored for one month after the study's conclusion as well. What researchers observed was that the children experienced substantial reductions in ADHD symptoms (hyperactivity, inattention, concentration, and eye-hand coordination) after four weeks of Pycnogenol administration.[447] One month after discontinuing the supplement, a relapse of symptoms occurred, which substantiated that the supplement was indeed the cause of reduced symptoms. Experts believe that the benefit of Pycnogenol is largely due to a balancing effect on total antioxidants, particularly increased glutathione (GSH) to oxidized glutathione (GSSG) ratios.[448,449] People with ADHD may have an impaired ability to combat the assault on neurons that results from oxidative stress, requiring extra support from a potent antioxidant like Pycnogenol.

Further research identified another mechanism behind the ADHD benefits of Pycnogenol. Forty-one people received Pycnogenol (1 mg/kg/day), and another sixteen people received a placebo. Overactivity of the neuronal system responsible for the production, storage, and release of norepinephrine was observed in people with ADHD when compared with healthy children. Furthermore, the researchers reported that higher norepinephrine levels directly corresponded with hyperactivity levels in ADHD children, and greater levels of adrenaline and norepinephrine were associated with increased amounts of oxidized glutathione (GSSG) in people with ADHD. Because glutathione is critical for protecting the brain from oxidative stress, the ratio of reduced glutathione (GSH) to oxidized glutathione is a key indicator of neuronal health. The study authors reported that Pycnogenol reduces the stress hormone adrenaline by over 26 percent and dopamine (a neurostimulant) by almost 11 percent, and increases the ratio of GSH to GSSG.[450] This balancing effect on stress hormones and antioxidant ratios results in decreased ADHD symptoms. Research regarding the benefits of Pycnogenol for people with ADHD is still emerging and requires additional larger and better controlled studies, but the results have been promising thus far, making it an option worth considering.

Phosphatidylserine

Phosphatidylserine (PS) is a naturally occurring phospholipid—a type of fat important to the structure and protection of cells—found in every cell in the human body. It is vital for brain function and the release of neurotransmitters is regulated by the amount of PS present in the membrane of neuronal cells. About half of your total PS is found in the brain—predominantly in the cell membranes of neurons. Its low molecular weight allows it to easily cross the blood-brain barrier—a filter that selectively allows substances into the brain. Once there, PS facilitates the storage, release, and activity of many neurotransmitters, heightens neuronal communication, and increases the fluidity of neuron cell membranes. Improved fluidity can improve cell signaling and function. It also stimulates the release of dopamine (influences mood and regulates physical sensations), improves glucose metabolism (fuels the brain), increases acetylcholine production (important for learning and memory), and elevates nerve growth factor activity (regulates growth, maintenance, abundance, and survival of neurons). When you consider the profound brain benefits of PS, it may be as essential for brain function as calcium is for bone strength.

Recognizing its importance in brain function, Japanese researchers set out to investigate its effect on ADHD symptoms in children aged four to fourteen who had not previously had any drug treatment for ADHD. During the two-month randomized and double-blind study, nineteen children received 200 mg of PS daily, whereas seventeen children in the control group received a placebo. The researchers observed that the children who received PS experienced significant improvements in short-term auditory memory, attention, and impulsivity.[451] One important fact with this study is that it identifies its source of PS as from soy lecithin. Many PS supplements are isolated from cow brain tissue, which is concerning considering mad cow disease.

A much larger study that included one hundred fifty children in Israel who were monitored for thirty weeks administered a product that combined PS with EPA and DHA (300 mg PS, 80 mg EPA, and 40 mg DHA). The advantage of taking PS directly linked to marine oils is that this combination ensures optimal delivery and performance. Children who received the PS/marine oil supplement experienced significant reductions in ADHD symptoms, particularly those with the hyperactive-impulsive subtype of ADHD.[452] This confirmed the findings of a previous study that demonstrated taking a combination PS and EPA/DHA supplement (300 mg PS, 250 mg EPA/DHA daily) eliminated

The Limbic System

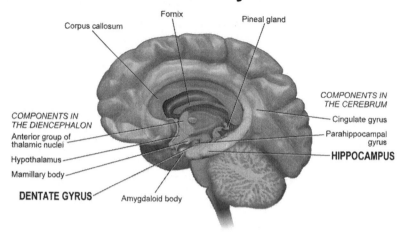

ADHD symptoms in 61 percent of children.[453] This is remarkable considering the study authors also included a control and a fish oil–only group that only experienced remission of symptoms in 14 and 33 percent of children respectively.

It is important to note that simply taking these two supplements (PS and EPA/DHA) separately will not likely be as effective. The fish oil must be directly linked (conjugated) to the phospholipid backbone—not just a simple mixture of fish oil and PS—for optimal effectiveness. Typical doses in studies range from 200 to 300 mg. With its promising research, PS—with or without fish oil—is worth considering as part of an overall ADHD management plan.[454]

Ginseng and Ginkgo Biloba

Both ginseng and ginkgo biloba (GB) act as cognitive activators, acting like stimulants but without the side effects of drugs. GB is one of the bestselling herbal supplements in Europe and the United States. The leaves of this tree contain flavonoids and terpenoids that act as antioxidants.[455,456] Antioxidants neutralize free radicals, preserving brain cells that may otherwise be damaged or destroyed. It also improves blood circulation—which may improve blood flow to the brain—and enhances dopamine signaling.[457,458,459] A special GB extract containing

24% flavonoids and 6% terpene lactone compounds (EGb 761) may also encourage the production of neural stem cells in the dentate gyrus and hippocampus—areas of the brain crucial for attention, memory, and learning.[460,461] Based on current research GB has great potential to improve cognitive fitness.

Ginseng is the generic term used for a variety of plants across the world that provide a human benefit. Interestingly, the plants called ginseng are not all from the same genus or family: Korean/Asian ginseng—*Panax ginseng;* American ginseng—*Panax quinquefolius*; Indian ginseng—*Withania somnifera*; Siberian ginseng—*Eleutherococcus senticosus*; Crown Prince ginseng—*Pseudostellaria heterophylla*; and Brazilian ginseng—*Pfaffia paniculata*. Traditionally, the two most popular varieties used for supplements—and true ginsengs—are Korean/Asian ginseng and American ginseng. These two species from the *Panax* genus contain ginsenosides or panaxosides, which are steroid glycosides. Steroid glycosides, or cardiac glycosides, dramatically influence the immune response, reduce inflammation, combat oxidative stress, protects against damage caused by stroke—particularly protecting neurons, and demonstrate promise in the fight against cancer.[462,463,464,465] Korean/Asian ginseng, also called red ginseng, is slightly stronger acting than American ginseng. The true ginsengs are known to increase brain performance, mental arithmetic abilities, and working memory, and perform similarly to serotonin and norepinephrine reuptake inhibitors (SNRIs).[466,467,468,469] Based on the clinical effects of ginseng, it is plausible that people with ADHD can benefit from supplementing with it.

A combination of GB and American ginseng improved a variety of ADHD symptoms, including social problems, hyperactivity, and impulsivity. Thirty-six children (aged three to seventeen years) were given capsules containing 200 mg of GB and 50 mg of American ginseng for four weeks on an empty stomach. Improvements in social behavior and hyperactivity-impulsivity were observed after only two weeks, with continued improvement through week four of using the supplement.[470]

Another study utilized GB standardized for terpenoids and isolated ginsenoside Rg3 from ginseng in mice. What the scientists found was that this combination reduced ADHD-like symptoms by reducing oxidative stress and enhancing dopamine and brain-derived neurotrophic factor (BDNF) signaling.[471] BDNF is vital to the survival of neurons, playing a role in the growth, differentiation (the process whereby a cell develops into a specialized cell to perform a specific function), and maintenance of these cells. It is also actively involved in synapses to improve cell-to-cell communication.

Preliminary research indicates that ginseng may be effective when administered alone. Two very small pilot studies that used Korean ginseng alone (250 mg, twice daily; or 1,000 mg, twice daily) demonstrated that ADHD symptoms of immaturity, inattention, and hyperactivity were reduced by the supplement.[472,473] Korean researchers reported similar effectiveness in a study that administered 1,000 mg of Korean ginseng (thirty-three children, ages six to fifteen years) twice daily.[474] Interestingly the study authors also reported that the children given Korean ginseng showed decreased theta/beta ratio as observed by quantitative electroencephalography. Higher theta/beta ratios are found in certain subtypes of ADHD, which suggests decreasing this ratio may reduce ADHD symptoms in some children.

GB has also been used alone in clinical trials investigating its effectiveness for ADHD. A preliminary study with only six people with ADHD demonstrated that GB improves hyperactivity, inattention, and immaturity symptoms.[475] A larger study (fifty children) administered 80 to 120 mg (80 mg/day for children under 30 lbs.; 120 mg/day for children over 30 lbs.) of GB or 20 to 30 mg of methylphenidate (again based on weight) for six weeks. Children in both groups experienced improvements in ADHD symptoms, but the GB group's symptom reduction was much less pronounced.[476] The same dosage was used in another study that also demonstrated improvement in ADHD symptoms with GB.[477] A pilot study (twenty children) evaluated the effect of EGb 761 (240 mg daily) on ADHD symptoms. After three to five weeks of taking the supplement core, ADHD symptoms were significantly improved.[478] Although the evidence is still preliminary, further examination of the benefits of GB for ADHD is warranted.

Both GB and ginseng require more evidence before they can be considered a viable alternative to stimulant medications. The preliminary research thus far has been promising and possibly suggests that taking them together will produce greater benefits. Until further larger scale research is completed, these two options should be considered after more viable alternatives like omega-3s and vitamins or minerals.

It would be unwise to try all of the above supplements at once. Instead, try one or two at a time, focusing on restoring any nutrient deficiencies first. If after a few to several weeks, you don't notice any difference, move on to another supplement. Always consult your doctor or pharmacist before using any supplements with medications to avoid sometimes serious interactions with medications. Supplements can be a worthwhile option if evidence-based decisions are made, high-quality supplements are chosen, and they are taken consistently enough to give them time to work.

Supplement Dosage Quick Reference	
OMEGA-3s *Particularly for children with learning difficulties*	*Pregnancy and lactation*: 1,000–1,500 mg DHA and 500–750 mg EPA daily
	Age 2 to 4: 500–750 mg DHA and 250–350 mg EPA
	Age 4 to 8: 750–1,000 mg DHA and 250–500 mg EPA
	Age 9 to 17: 1,250–1,500 mg DHA and 750–1,000 EPA
	18+: 1,500–2,000 mg DHA and 1,000–1,250 mg EPA

VITAMIN D	2,000 IU or dosage recommended by physician
IRON *Particularly for children with inattentive subtype; or children with sleep disturbances or restless leg syndrome*	5 mg/kg daily; or 80 mg daily *Doses exceeding 40–45 mg daily should only be taken under the care of a physician.*
ZINC *Particularly for children with hyperactive-impulsive subtype*	1mg/kg daily *Doses exceeding the upper limit daily should only be taken under the care of a physician.*
MAGNESIUM	Citrate: 54.5–560 w/B6: 6–100 mg MgT: 350–2,000 mg
PYCNOGENOL	1 mg/kg daily
PHOSPHATIDYL-SERINE *Particularly for children with hyperactive-impulsive subtype*	200–300 mg daily
GINKGO BILOBA + AMERICAN GINSENG	Ginkgo biloba: 200–250 mg daily; 80 mg/day for children under 30 lbs. or 120 mg/day for children over 30 lbs. American ginseng: 50 mg daily
GINKGO BILOBA	>30 lbs.: 80 mg daily <30 lbs.: 120 mg daily
KOREAN GINSENG	250–1,000 mg, twice daily

Essential Oils

Essential oils can profoundly influence mood, mental performance, and brain function. They simultaneously work on the physical, mental, emotional, and spiritual levels of wellness. Some essential oils balance neurotransmitters in the brain by acting on the pathways that create, release, balance, and control neurotransmitters. Others influence the function and activity of key systems (nervous, endocrine) that may reduce ADHD symptoms. At the very least, they can encourage a more relaxed state of body and mind, which allows the body to more rapidly correct imbalances and heal. Once you experience the power of essential oils, you are likely to incorporate them into your daily life more regularly.

A great deal of research suggests that imbalances of neurotransmitters and hormones (caused by genetics or abnormal brain structure and function) influences ADHD symptoms. Dopamine and norepinephrine work in tandem with glutamate to maintain a tightly controlled balance of neurotransmitters. Serotonin is another neurotransmitter that is emerging as important in brain function and ADHD due to its influence on mood, memory, learning, social behavior, attention, and regulation of dopamine signaling. If this delicate balance of neurotransmitters is disrupted, a person can feel understimulated, inattentive, impulsive, and hyperactive. Stimulant drugs work by modifying neurotransmitter levels to help the person feel more "normal." Scientific research has revealed that some essential oils can also influence these neurotransmitters and hormone levels to modify behavior, attention, and activity levels.

- Inhalation of eucalyptus essential oil (*E. globulus*) increases the release of dopamine by almost 2.5 times in rats.[479] The study authors concluded that inhalation of essential oils stimulates dopamine-releasing cells to release dopamine, which may affect brain functions involved in attention, reward, and mood.
- Lemon essential oil influences dopamine and serotonin activity in mice when inhaled.[480] The researchers found that lemon essential oil activated pathways related to reducing anxiety and depression, which suggests if a child has ADHD and anxiety or depression lemon essential oil may be worth incorporating.
- Inhalation of lavender essential oil balances serotonin activity in the brain and reduces excess serotonin levels that may cause serotonin syndrome (when excess serotonin is released and remains in the brain, causing agitation, diarrhea, hallucinations, rapid heartbeat, high

blood pressure, and loss of coordination).[481] Again, this would be most beneficial with those who have anxiety or depression in addition to ADHD. Lavender essential oil also binds to GABA receptors on cells to reduce excitatory activity that causes anxiety, panic, and fear, possibly by balancing serotonin and norepinephrine levels.[482,483]

In addition to influencing neurotransmitters, some essential oils directly influence symptoms of ADHD. Through modulating central nervous system activity, arousal levels, and focusing the mind, these essential oils may improve core symptoms of ADHD when inhaled or applied.

- A very small study (three adolescents, age fourteen to sixteen years) investigated the effect of a German chamomile supplement on ADHD symptoms. The study author concluded that taking tablets containing 100 mg alpha-bisabolol (extract 1:4.0 with ethanol 96%) and 190 mg of German chamomile essential oil three times daily for four weeks proved slightly effective in reducing ADHD symptoms (hyperactivity, inattention, and immaturity).[484] The study author attributed this benefit to reduced serotonin and norepinephrine reuptake.
- Inhalation of bay laurel essential oil improved careful concentration and attention to task performance— critical to reading, writing, learning, and social behavior.[485] Study participants inhaled bay laurel scent for forty-five minutes while performing the task. It may be beneficial to place a couple of drops on a diffuser necklace or in a personal inhaler for your child to inhale when needed during school.
- Inhalation of peppermint essential oil enhances attention and arousal while performing clerical tasks.[486] Scientists concluded that diffusing peppermint essential oil during a typing test increased speed and accuracy and the ability to alphabetize.

- Vetiver increases visual-discrimination task performance (critical to reading, writing, learning, and social behavior) when inhaled.[487] Vetiver may benefit ADHD symptoms by calming and focusing the mind. Remarkably, it only required 0.25 mcg (a fraction of a drop) of vetiver essential oil to produce results.
- Orange-peel essential oil is up to 95.4% d-limonene. This terpene compound is a potent antioxidant that prevents free-radical damage linked to disrupted cellular communication and the premature destruction of cells.[488] It also preserves the body's stores of reduced glutathione (GSH) and encourages the body to produce GSH.[489] Glutathione is a key antioxidant in brain detoxification and helps capture and remove heavy metals from the body. In addition, the metabolites of citrus terpene compounds (like limonene) trigger the release of neurotransmitters (dopamine, noradrenaline, serotonin) in rats.[490] Orange essential oil may relieve ADHD symptoms by protecting brain cells and removing heavy metals that could interfere with neuronal communication.

Another emerging aspect of essential oils in relation to ADHD is their ability to influence brain electrical activity. The image on the next page demonstrates how inhalation of frankincense affects brain waves and electrical activity. After the administration of frankincense essential oil, an increase in 13–15 Hz beta and a substantial normalization of 21–23 Hz beta in absolute power (compared to peer database) was observed. This correlates with neurophysiological markers of improved attention due to decreased hypervigilance (an abnormal state of enhanced sensory sensitivity to external stimuli accompanied by anxiety) and mind racing, as well as a balanced stress response. These remarkable images demonstrate that inhalation of frankincense essential oil increases focus and attention—making it useful for ADHD—most likely due to stabilization of the limbic system.

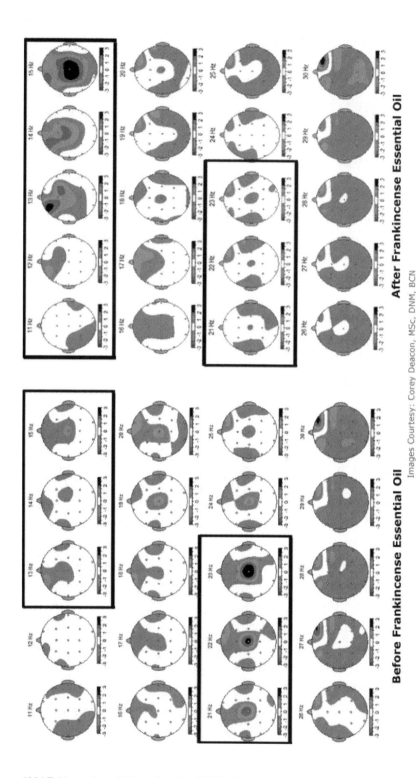

After Frankincense Essential Oil

Before Frankincense Essential Oil

Images Courtesy: Corey Deacon, MSc, DNM, BCN

Based on the above research, and correlating these findings with clinical experience, the following essential oil blend may be helpful in reducing ADHD symptoms. In a 15 ml bottle add the following in the order provided:

- 10 drops of frankincense essential oil
- 3 drops of vetiver essential oil
- 5 drops of lavender essential oil
- 6 drops of orange essential oil
- 3 drops of eucalyptus (*E. globulus*) essential oil (omit eucalyptus in children under three years of age)
- 3 drops of peppermint (omit peppermint in children under three years of age)
- Fill the rest of the bottle with carrier oil (grapeseed, fractionated-coconut oil, or sweet almond oil are good choices)

Once the blend is created, put a few drops in an essential oil inhaler, diffuser necklace, or on a tissue and inhale as needed; and/or apply 1 drop to the back of the neck, base of the skull, and crown of the head two to three times daily.

Conclusion

There are a number of natural options available to reduce ADHD symptoms and improve overall quality of life. Supplementation requires patience, persistence, and experimentation to discover the best option for your children. Essential oils can have rapid effects, but must be used frequently to maintain results due to their volatility. Taking supplements in conjunction with essential oils is more likely to yield positive and sustainable results. When choosing your supplements, focus on insufficiencies or deficiencies in nutrients first. Once these nutrients have been restored to optimum levels, consider adding additional supplements one to two at a time and monitoring the results. Try each new supplement for about four weeks to determine its effectiveness. Evidence-based natural options may be the key element missing in your ADHD management plan.

6

MUSIC AND OCCUPATIONAL THERAPY

On the fringe of traditional treatment options for ADHD are two additional therapies—music and occupational therapy. Both therapies involve trained therapists who work with individuals that have special needs such as mental, physical, developmental, or emotional restrictions. These therapies should not be easily dismissed and have merit worth considering as part of an overall treatment program. The goal of each therapy is to address emotional, cognitive, and social issues, and to help people of all ages live productive and satisfying lives.

Music Therapy

Music therapy employs the evidence-based use of music interventions to enhance wellness, reduce the negative effects of stress, encourage appropriate expression of feelings, improve memory, and foster communication. Credentialed professionals who have completed an approved music-therapy program use music to address the physical, emotional, cognitive, and social needs of individual clients. Based on the individual's needs, therapy may include creating, listening to, singing, or moving to music or doing some combination of these.

The connection between music and physical, mental, emotional, and spiritual health has been recognized for centuries. Pythagoras, Plato, and Aristotle each taught that music affects both health and behavior. Indigenous cultures from all over the world incorporated music into their healing arts. But it wasn't until the 1960s and the 1970s that scientists really began to investigate the healing power of music in clinical trials. These trials demonstrated that strong rhythmic music pieces can affect heart rate and breathing, reduce muscle tension, relieve pain, encourage deep relaxation, and promote the release of endorphins.[491,492,493,494,495] Rapidly developing technology (like brain-imaging techniques) and mounting scientific evidence has armed researchers with the ability to identify how music affects brain activity and heals and strengthens the brain. Indeed, few things have the ability to activate and affect the brain as profoundly as music.

Music therapy may improve the auditory abilities of children with ADHD, which may improve attention and learning. Some research has found that children with ADHD have reduced volumes of the auditory cortex.[496] Reduced auditory processing abilities is strongly associated with attentional and literacy problems. If you can't hear properly, you have a tendency to feel disconnected, and it often results in poor academic performance. Fortunately, evidence suggests that music therapy may encourage regeneration and adaptation of the auditory cortex.[497,498] Restoration of hearing abilities can profoundly influence academic performance and social behaviors. If learning disabilities are present with ADHD, music therapy is an excellent option.

For children with ADHD, music therapy fosters improved attention, focus, and social skills, while simultaneously reducing hyperactivity. Music benefits the ADHD brain partly because it provides structure and enhances circuitry. Rhythmic music provides structure that is soothing to the ADHD brain. It activates and connects the right and left hemispheres of the brain, which improves overall brain function. In addition, it triggers synaptic firing that increases dopamine levels in the brain.[499,500] Music affects everyone and can arouse deep feelings. These feelings are likely the result of increased release of endorphins, neurotransmitters, and hormones that may explain why music is placed in high value across all cultures.

Very little published research reports the direct benefits or music therapy for ADHD; however, statements from parents, teachers, and clinicians suggest it is valuable for the ADHD brain. It is also well-known that music therapy modulates some of the key irregularities seen in ADHD brain function. Music engages the auditory, visual, and tactile senses, which activates and stimulates areas of the brain that other modalities may not. The multisensory experience provided by music helps organize the sensory systems, balances sensory responses, and enhances self-regulation. When a person listens to music, it stimulates the reward centers of the brain, which in turn can reinforce positive social behavior and reduce self-stimulatory responses. Music rhythms can also be used as an external timekeeper to improve coordination and movement (motor skills). These are just a few of the ways that music therapy could benefit the ADHD brain.

Unlike other therapies that may affect sexes, ages, and subtypes of ADHD differently, evidence suggests that music therapy is effective regardless of age, sex, intelligence, or background.[501] Reductions in a range of ADHD symptoms (impulsiveness, restlessness, and hyperactivity) and improvements in synchronized finger tapping (used to measure auditory detection) to an auditory rhythm have been observed in children listening to music.[502] Despite a lack of evidence-based research directly related to ADHD, countless user experiences and compelling evidence regarding how music affects the brain make music therapy a valuable adjunct therapy option.

LEFT BRAIN	RIGHT BRAIN
Controls Right Side of Body	Controls Left Side of Body
Logic and Rationality	Imagination/Visualization
Mathematics & Science	Creativity
Analysis	Intuition
Sequencing	Calmness
Alertness	Holistic Thinking
Language	Arts (Motor Skill)
Facts	Non-verbal
Judgement	Feelings
Short-term Memory	Fantasy-based
Computation	Long-term Memory
Detail Oriented	Symbols and Images
Order/Pattern Based	Daydreaming

Classical music does not contain lyrics, which allows the listener to avoid the distraction of attempting to understand lyrics. Remarkably, scientists have discovered that listening to classical music modulates genes responsible for brain function.

Specifically, classical music enhances gene activity involved in the release and transport of dopamine, synaptic transmission, learning and memory, and reduces activity of genes involved in brain degeneration.[503] A number of classical songs are frequently used to benefit the ADHD brain, improve focus, speech, and quality of sleep. These classical pieces contain patterns, details, and dimensions (rhythmic, structural, temporal, and mathematical) that build the brain (advances speech and language skills), stimulate the inner ear (beneficial for children with learning or auditory difficulties), modify brain waves (improves focus and concentration), soothe overactive minds, and improves impulse control and comprehension.

- Wolfgang Amadeus Mozart: "Violin Concerto, No. 3, G-major, K.216"
- Ludwig van Beethoven: "Emperor Concerto for Piano, No. 5"
- Antonio Vivaldi: "The Four Seasons"
- Wolfgang Amadeus Mozart: "Symphony No. 40 in G Minor"
- Johann Sebastian Bach: "Brandenburg Concertos"
- Peter Ilyich Tchaikovsky: "Concerto for Piano No. 1"
- George Frideric Handel: "Water Music"
- Johann Pachelbel: "Canon in D"
- Johannes Brahms: "Concerto for Violin, D Major"

Occupational Therapy

Like music therapy, occupational therapy is an individualized therapy that helps people with physical, sensory, or cognitive disabilities become as independent as possible and enjoy a rewarding and fulfilling life. Occupational therapists help people participate in everyday occupations (normal activities they want or need to do). For example, an occupation for a child would be daily activities, playing, and school performance. Occupational therapy primarily focuses on fine motor, visual-perception, cognitive, and sensory-processing skills. Its ultimate goal is to help people of all ages who need special assistance to realize an improved quality of life.

Children with ADHD often struggle with tasks such as handwriting, organization, and other everyday tasks at home and school. It can be overwhelming to the parent of these children to balance career, family, religious, educational, and other responsibilities, along with finding adequate time to focus on improving their child's task performance. Occupational therapists can fill this role and help your child strengthen executive function skills and self-regulation, better manage time, and improve organization skills to perform better on ordinary tasks. In other words, they will help them discover strategies to overcome some of the limitations and difficulties they experience because of ADHD.

As part of occupational therapy, the therapist will do the following:

- Evaluate how ADHD is affecting your child's performance at home and school
- Identify goals that can help the child succeed
- Recommend an individualized plan that addresses any physical, emotional, or behavioral roadblocks caused by ADHD
- Utilize sensory integration—how people respond to information provided by the senses—to adapt the environment to decrease distractions caused by visual, auditory, or tactile stimulation

Children with ADHD are not as able to adapt to daily sensory stimulation from their external environment as their non-ADHD peers. They can be easily distracted or disturbed by a sound or movement, making it harder to pay attention to their parents or teacher. To them, small noises may be loud and obnoxious, or it could be the opposite—that normal sensory stimuli from the environment could seem faded and obscure. Either way, troublesome behaviors at school and home can occur as they withdraw from or seek out sensory stimulation. An inability to adapt to sensory stimuli is often caused by underlying sensory and neurological issues that can be addressed by occupational therapy.

Signs of Sensory-Processing Difficulties	
Overresponsiveness (Hypersensitivities):	✓ Sudden, high-pitched or loud noises ✓ Easily distracted by background noises ✓ Poor balance, falls often ✓ Dislikes crowds or avoids standing in close proximity to others ✓ Avoids hugs or cuddling with familiar adults ✓ Fearful of climbing or falling; dislikes feet being off the ground ✓ Startled easily by surprise touch
Underresponsiveness (Hyposensitivities):	✓ Constant need to touch people or textures ✓ Thrill seeking ✓ Fidgety, unable to sit still ✓ Likes to spin and jump ✓ Uncoordinated ✓ Extremely high tolerance for pain ✓ Inadvertently harms other children or pets when playing (doesn't know his or her own strength) ✓ Doesn't respect personal space of others

Occupational therapy sessions engage the three basic sensory systems: tactile—controls the sense of touch; vestibular—controls the sensations of gravity and movement; and proprioceptive—controls the awareness of the body in space in relation to position, motion, and equilibrium. Techniques are employed during occupational therapy sessions that are tailored to the child's needs in each of these basic sensory systems. For example, techniques such as deep pressure, climbing while wearing a weighted vest, light skin brushing, or working with an exercise ball may be employed. The goal is to increase the person's awareness of these sensations through activating the nervous system and improving the brain's plasticity and adaptability to sensory stimuli.

Temple University researchers investigated whether ADHD symptoms could be decreased by addressing underlying sensory and neurological difficulties. Eighty-eight children were included in the study, all of which were taking medication for ADHD. The study authors divided the children into two groups: sixty-three children participated in forty one-hour occupational therapy sessions that focused on sensory interventions; whereas twenty-five children did not. At the conclusion of the six-month study, the researchers noted significant improvements in sensory integration, which corresponded with significant declines in ADHD symptoms.[504] Other research suggests that occupational therapy positively influences brain waves to increase the attention span of children with ADHD, and improves social interactions with peers.[505,506,507]

Another study included twenty children of varying subtypes of ADHD who also experienced sensory integration difficulties (half also had developmental coordination disorder—a disorder marked by clumsiness in otherwise healthy children). A specific family-centered protocol (parent and teacher education, behavioral management, sensory integration, classroom environment adaptation, and additional treatments to address developmental and functional difficulties), involving twelve weekly contacts, was conducted for three months. About half of the children—from various subtypes—experienced reduced ADHD symptoms by the completion of the study.[508] While the research is still very preliminary, occupational therapy may be a good option for children who experience sensory difficulties.

Conclusion

Music therapy is low cost if you simply purchase the mentioned classical music and have your child listen for at least twenty minutes daily. A music therapist can also be of great help in selecting the appropriate time and types of music for your child. Occupational therapy will cost for the therapist's time and each visit, but many therapists are willing to train parents how to do some of the therapy at home. In addition, special tools (body socks, resistance tunnel, pressure bed sheets, etc.) can also be purchased to retrain the nervous system to respond more appropriately to sensations. There is very little to lose and a lot to possibly gain by incorporating either of these therapies into your overall ADHD management plan.

7

CONCLUSION

Hopefully by now you have a better understanding of the complexity of ADHD and what your child may be experiencing, or a more complete understanding of all the factors that influence your own symptoms. The complex possibilities that influence ADHD make a comprehensive and fluid management plan a must. All options that have the possibility of improving the ability of a person with ADHD to function better in society and have a rewarding and fulfilling life should be considered, with emphasis on the least harmful options first.

Stimulant drugs are the most common treatment prescribed for ADHD, but they aren't the only answer, nor are they always effective. Up to 30 percent of people with ADHD do not respond to them. In addition, they have side effects and risks to consider—some serious. Behavior therapy is a great option to reinforce positive behaviors and reduce negative learned responses. It is effective where medications are not. Have the courage to question medications that are prescribed and really determine the benefits versus the risks of any medication.

School doesn't have to be one of the most challenging situations facing your child. A few reasonable adaptations and accommodations can significantly increase your child's success in school. Make sure to partner with all people involved in his or her education, including the teacher, counselor, and administrators. If you don't act as advocate for your child in his or her schooling, no one else likely will.

Nutrition is the foundation of all health. Those with chronic conditions generally have specific nutrient requirements or deficiencies or both. If deficiencies or insufficiencies of nutrients exist, restore these nutrients to optimal levels with better eating. Don't power your body with garbage fuel and expect it to perform at its best. Give it the best fuel available, which will encourage the optimal functioning of key body systems. Empty calories (sugar, refined carbohydrates) should be reduced significantly and replaced with wholesome foods. Food sensitivities should be identified and mitigated. Rebuild gut health and restore intestinal balance, making sure to support the good guys in your microbiome. As you provide your body with a steady stream of nutrients, cells will work more efficiently, leading to healthier tissues, organs, and organs systems that thrive.

Dietary supplements and essential oils can be a crucial partner in your overall ADHD management plan. Choose evidence-based supplements based on your child's needs. Chapter 5 outlines supplements and essential oils that have the most promise for a positive result. More importantly the subtypes that are most likely to respond to those options are identified. Focus on supplements that restore nutrient deficiencies not corrected by diet first, then give a supplement or two a try and carefully monitor the results. Essential oils can profoundly influence overall well-being, often just by inhaling these powerful molecules. You may find the knockout punch you are seeking in a carefully selected supplement or essential oil.

Enjoy music frequently, particularly classical music that deeply affects the brain and its function. Connecting both hemispheres of the brain can produce surprising and remarkable results as history demonstrates. Arizona congresswoman Gabby Giffords lost the ability to speak due to a gunshot wound to the left side of her brain. Music therapy is partially credited for restoring that ability. Occupational therapy, like behavioral therapy, can benefit aspects of yours or your child's life that medications won't, such as organization and self-regulation skills. It is an effective way to enhance fine-motor skills, sensory processing, visual perception, and cognitive skills. Either therapy is undoubtedly worth a try.

Be patient, be adaptive, and be persistent. Much of what you will learn will come as the result of trial and error. What works for one person with ADHD may not work for another. But by incorporating natural approaches, you are giving yourself or your child a better chance of success and improved quality of life. Natural options are all about restoring balance and optimal function of cells, organs, and body systems. This puts your body in better condition to manage ADHD. Simply relying on medication alone is not a long-term solution. When the medication is discontinued, symptoms are highly likely to reoccur. Now is the time to take what you have learned, apply it to your situation, and move forward with faith that it is possible to *Beat ADHD Naturally.*

*****

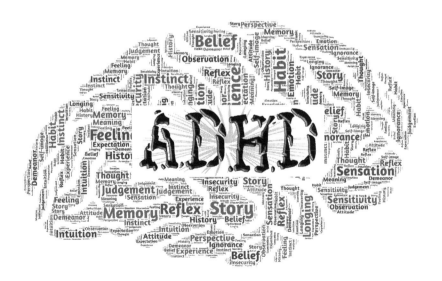

REFERENCES

[1] U.S. Centers for Disease Control and Prevention. Attention-Deficit/Hyperactivity Disorder (ADHD). Data & Statistics. Available at: http://www.cdc.gov/ncbddd/adhd/data.html.

[2] Morton WA, Stockton GG. Methylphenidate Abuse and Psychiatric Side Effects. Prim Care Companion J Clin Psychiatry. 2000 Oct;2(5):159–164.

[3] Burt SA. Are there shared environmental influences on attention-deficit/hyperactivity disorder? Reply to Wood, Buitelaar, Rijsdijk, Asherson, and Kuntsi [corrected] (2010). Psychol Bull. 2010 May;136(3):341–3.

[4] Burt SA. Rethinking environmental contributions to child and adolescent psychopathology: a meta-analysis of shared environmental influences. Psychol Bull. 2009 Jul;135(4):608–37.

[5] Volkow ND, Wang GJ, Kollins SH, et al. Evaluating Dopamine Reward Pathway in ADHD: Clinical Implications. JAMA. 2009;302(10):1084–1091.

[6] Volkow ND, Wang GJ, Kollins SH, et al. Evaluating Dopamine Reward Pathway in ADHD. JAMA. 2009 Sep 9; 302(10): 1084–1091.

[7] Blum K, Chen ALC, Braveman ER, et al. Attention-deficit-hyperactivity disorder and reward deficiency syndrome. Neuropsychiatr Dis Treat. 2008 Oct;4(5):893–918.

[8] U.S. Centers for Disease Control and Prevention. Attention-Deficit/Hyperactivity Disorder (ADHD). Available at: http://www.cdc.gov/ncbddd/adhd/data.html.

[9] U.S. Centers for Disease Control and Prevention. NCH Data Brief: Attention Deficit Hyperactivity Disorder Among Children Aged 5–17 Years in the United States, 1998–2009. 2011 Aug. Available at: http://www.cdc.gov/nchs/data/databriefs/db70.htm.

[10] Barkley RA, Fischer M, Smallish L, et al. The persistence of attention-deficit/hyperactivity disorder into young adulthood as a function of reporting source and definition of disorder. J Abnorm Psychol 2002;111:279–289.

[11] Ebejer JL, Medland SE, van der Werf J, et al. Attention deficit hyperactivity disorder in Australian adults: prevalence, persistence, conduct problems and disadvantage. PLoS One 2012;7:e47404.

[12] Faraone SV, Biederman J, Mick E. The age-dependent decline of attention deficit hyperactivity disorder: a meta-analysis of follow-up studies. Psychol Med 2006;36:159–165.

[13] Lara C, Fayyad J, de Graaf R, et al. Childhood predictors of adult attention-deficit/hyperactivity disorder: results from the World

Health Organization World Mental Health Survey Initiative. Biol Psychiatry 2009;65:46–54.

[14] U.S. Centers for Disease Control and Prevention. Attention-Deficit/Hyperactivity Disorder (ADHD). Available at: http://www.cdc.gov/ncbddd/adhd/data.html.

[15] Fayyad J, de Graaf R, Kessler R, et al. Cross-national prevalence and correlates of adult attention-deficit hyperactivity disorder. Br J Psychiatry 2007;190:402–409.

[16] Wolinsky H. Disease mongering and drug marketing. EMBO Rep. 2005 Jul;6(7):612–614.

[17] Metha ES. Why self-regulation does not work: resolving prescription corruption caused by excessive gift-giving by pharmaceutical manufacturers. Food Drug Law J. 2008;63(4):799–821.

[18] Wall LL, Brown D. The high cost of free lunch. Obstet Gynecol. 2007 Jul;110(1):169–73.

[19] Collins J. Professionalism and physician interactions with industry. J Am Coll Radiol. 2006 May;3(5):325–32.

[20] U.S. Centers for Disease Control and Prevention. Attention-Deficit/Hyperactivity Disorder (ADHD). Available at: http://www.cdc.gov/ncbddd/adhd/guidelines.html.

[21] Visser SN, Lesesne CA, Perou R. National estimates and factors associated with medication treatment for childhood attention-deficit/hyperactivity disorder. Pediatrics. 2007 Feb;119 Suppl 1:S99–106.

[22] LeFever GB, Arcona AP, Antonuccio DO. National estimates and factors associated with medication treatment for childhood attention-deficit/hyperactivity disorder. Pediatrics. 2007;119(suppl 1):S99–S106.

[23] Cajochen C, Frey S, Anders D, et al. Evening exposure to a light-emitting diodes (LED)-backlit computer screen affects circadian physiology and cognitive performance. J Appl Physiol. 2011 May;110(5):1432–38.

[24] Wood B, Rea MS, Plitnick B, et al. Light level and duration of exposure determine the impact of self-luminous tablets on melatonin suppression. Appl Ergonomics. 2013 Mar;44(2):237–40.

[25] Kooij JJ, Bijlenga D. The circadian rhythm in adult attention-deficit/hyperactivity disorder: current state of affairs. Expert Rev Neurother. 2013 Oct;13(10):1107–16.

[26] Rybak YE, McNeely HE, Mackenzie BE, et al. Seasonality and circadian preference in adult attention-deficit/hyperactivity disorder: clinical and neuropsychological correlates. Compr Psychiatry. 2007 Nov–Dec;48(6):562–71.

[27] Radesky JS, Silverstein M, Zuckerman B, et al. Infant Self-Regulation and Early Childhood Media Exposure. Pediatrics. 2014 May;133(5):e1772–78.

[28] Page AS, Cooper AR, Griew P, et al. Children's Screen Viewing is Related to Psychological Difficulties Irrespective of Physical Activity. Pediatrics. 2010 Oct;126(5):e1011–7.

[29] Swing EL, Gentile DA, Anderson CA, et al. Television and Video Game Exposure and the Development of Attention Problems. Pediatrics. 2010 Jun;126(2):214–21.

[30] Gottschalk A, Flocke SA. Time Spent in Face-to-Face Patient Care and Work Outside the Examination Room. Ann Fam Med. 2005 Nov; 3(6): 488–493.

[31] Fulton BD, Scheffler RM, Hinshaw SP. State Variation in Increased ADHD Prevalence: Links to NCLB School Accountability and State Medication Laws. Psychiatr Serv. 2015 Oct;66(10):1074–82.

[32] Bokhari FA, Schneider H. School accountability laws and the consumption of psychostimulants. J Health Econ. 2011 Mar;30(2):355–72.

[33] Faraone SV, Perlis RH, Doyle AE, et al. Molecular genetics of attention-deficit/hyperactivity disorder. Biol Psychiatry 2005;57:1313–23.

[34] Burt SA. Rethinking environmental contributions to child and adolescent psychopathology: a meta-analysis of shared environmental influences. Psychol Bull 2009;135:608–637.

[35] Thapar A, Cooper M, Eyre O, et al. What have we learnt about the causes of ADHD? J Child Psychol Psychiatry. 2013 Jan;54(1):3–16.

[36] Zhang L, Chang S, Li S, et al. ADHDgene: a genetic database for attention deficit hyperactivity disorder. Nucleic Acids Res. 2012 Jan;40(Database issue):D1003–D1009.

[37] Gizer IR, Ficks C, Waldman ID. Candidate gene studies of ADHD: a meta-analytic review. Hum. Genet. 2009;126:51–90.

[38] Zhou K, Dempfle A, Arcos-Burgos M, et al. Meta-analysis of genome-wide linkage scans of attention deficit hyperactivity disorder. Am. J. Med. Genet. B Neuropsychiatr. Genet. 2008;147B:1392–1398.

[39] Neale BM, Medland SE, Ripke S, et al. Meta-analysis of genome-wide association studies of attention-deficit/hyperactivity disorder. J. Am. Acad. Child Adolesc. Psychiatry. 2010;49:884–897.

[40] Elia J, Gai X, Xie HM, et al. Rare structural variants found in attention-deficit hyperactivity disorder are preferentially associated with neurodevelopmental genes. Mol. Psychiatry. 2010;15:637–646.

[41] Williams NM, Zaharieva I, Martin A, et al. Rare chromosomal deletions and duplications in attention-deficit hyperactivity disorder: a genome-wide analysis. Lancet. 2010;376:1401–1408.

[42] Lesch KP, Selch S, Renner TJ, et al. Genome-wide copy number variation analysis in attention-deficit/hyperactivity disorder: association with neuropeptide Y gene dosage in an extended pedigree. Mol. Psychiatry. 2011;16:491–503.

[43] Brookes K, Xu X, Chen W, et al. The analysis of 51 genes in DSM-IV combined type attention deficit hyperactivity disorder: association signals in DRD4, DAT1 and 16 other genes. Mol. Psychiatry. 2006;11:934–953.

[44] Johansson S, Halleland H, Halmoy A, et al. Genetic analyses of dopamine related genes in adult ADHD patients suggest an association with the DRD5–microsatellite repeat, but not with DRD4 or SLC6A3 VNTRs. Am. J. Med. Genet. B Neuropsychiatr. Genet. 2008;147B:1470–1475.

[45] Tahir E, Yazgan Y, Cirakoglu B, et al. Association and linkage of DRD4 and DRD5 with attention deficit hyperactivity disorder (ADHD) in a sample of Turkish children. Mol Psychiatry. 2000 Jul;5(4):396–404.

[46] Bakker SC, van der Meulen EM, Oteman N, et al. DAT1, DRD4, and DRD5 polymorphisms are not associated with ADHD in Dutch families. Am J Med Genet B Neuropsychiatr Genet. 2005 Jan 5;132B(1):50–2.

[47] Henrichsen CN, Chaignat E, Reymond A. Copy number variants, diseases and gene expression Hum Mol Genet. 2009;18(R1):R1–R8.

[48] Shlien A, Malkin D. Copy number variations and cancer. Genome Med. 2009 Jun 16;1(6):62.

[49] Willyard C. Copy number variations' effect on drug response still overlooked. Nature Medicine. 2015 Mar;21(3):206.

[50] He Y, Hoskins JM, McLeod HL. Copy Number Variants in pharmacogenetic genes. Trends Mol Med. 2011 May; 17(5):244–251.

[51] Thomas AG, Dennis A, Bandettini PA, et al. The Effects of Aerobic Activity on Brain Structure. Front Psychol. 2012;3:86.

[52] Holzel BK, Carmody J, Vangel M, et al. Mindfulness practice leads to increases in regional brain gray matter density. Psychiatry Res. 2011 Jan 30;191(1):36–43.

[53] Maguire EA, Woollett K, Spiers HJ. London taxi drivers and bus drivers: a structural MRI and neuropsychological analysis. Hippocampus. 2006;16(12):1091–101.

[54] Bremner JD. Traumatic stress: effects on the brain. Dialogues Clin Neurosci. 2006 Dec;8(4):445–461.

[55] Davenport ND, Karatekin C, White T, et al. Differential fractional anisotropy abnormalities in adolescents with ADHD or schizophrenia. Psychiatry Res. 2010;181:193–98.

[56] Ellison-Wright I, Ellison-Wright Z, Bullmore E. Structural brain change in Attention Deficit Hyperactivity Disorder identified by meta-analysis. BMC Psychiatry. BMC Psychiatry. 2008 Jun 30;8:51.

[57] Kobel M, Bechtel N, Specht K, et al. Structural and functional imaging approaches in attention deficit/hyperactivity disorder: does the temporal lobe play a key role? Psychiatry Res. 2010;183:230–36.

[58] Ivanov I, Bansal R, Hao X, et al. Morphological abnormalities of the thalamus in youths with attention deficit hyperactivity disorder. Am J Psychiatry. 2010;167:397–408.

[59] Nakao T, Radua J, Rubia K, et al. Gray matter volume abnormalities in ADHD: voxel-based meta-analysis exploring the effects of age and stimulant medication. Am J Psychiatry. 2011;168:1154–63.

[60] Pavuluri MN, Yang S, Kamineni K, et al. Diffusion tensor imaging study of white matter fiber tracts in pediatric bipolar disorder and attention-deficit/hyperactivity disorder. Biol Psychiatry. 2009;65:586–93.

[61] Shaw P, Lerch J, Greenstein D, et al. Longitudinal mapping of cortical thickness and clinical outcome in children and adolescents with attention-deficit/hyperactivity disorder. Arch Gen Psychiatry. 2006;63: 540–49.

[62] Shaw P, Malek M, Watson B, et al. Development of cortical surface area and gyrification in attention-deficit/hyperactivity disorder. Biol Psychiatry. 2012;2:191–197.

[63] Shaw P, Eckstand K, Sharp W, et al. Attention-deficit/hyperactivity disorder is characterized by a delay in cortical maturation. PNAS. 2007 Oct;104(9):19649–54.

[64] Batty MJ, Liddle EB, Pitiot A, et al. Cortical gray matter in attention-deficit/hyperactivity disorder: a structural magnetic resonance imaging study. J Am Acad Child Adolesc Psychiatry. 2010 Mar;49(3):229–38.

[65] Nakao T, Radua J, Rubia K, et al. Gray Matter Volume Abnormalities in ADHD: Voxel-Based Meta-Analysis Exploring the Effects of Age and Stimulant Medication. Am J Psychiatry. 2011;168(11):1154–63.

[66] Ames BJ, Claus ED, Depue BE, et al. Gray and White matter differences in young adults with ADHD. Available at: http://spot.colorado.edu/~burgessg/pdf/Ames_HBM2006_ADHD_V BM.pdf.

[67] Vaidya CJ. Neurodevelopmental Abnormalities in ADHD. Curr Top Behav Neurosci. 2012; 9: 49–66.

[68] Sowell ER, Thompson PM, Welcome SE, et al. Cortical abnormalities in children and adolescents with attention-deficit hyperactivity disorder. Lancet. 2003;362:1699–1707.

[69] Silk TJ, Vance A, Rinehart N, et al. White-matter abnormalities in attention deficit hyperactivity disorder: a diffusion tensor imaging study. Hum Brain Mapp. 2009 Sep;30(9):2757–65.

[70] Nagel BJ, Bathula D, Herting M, et al. Altered white matter microstructure in children with attention-deficit/hyperactivity disorder. J Am Acad Child Adolesc Psychiatry. 2011 Mar;50(3):283–92.

[71] Wang Y, Horst KK, Kronenberger WG, et al. White matter abnormalities associated with disruptive behavior disorder in adolescents with and without attention-deficit/hyperactivity disorder. Psychiatry Res. 2012 Jun 30;202(3):245–51.

[72] Onnink AM, Zwiers MP, Hoogman M, et al. Deviant white matter structure in adults with attention-deficit/hyperactivity disorder points to aberrant myelination and affects neuropsychological performance. Prog Neuropsychopharmacol Biol Psychiatry. 2015 Dec 3;63:14–22.

[73] Ellison-Wright I, Ellison-Wright Z, Bullmore E. Structural brain change in Attention Deficit Hyperactivity Disorder identified by meta-analysis. BMC Psychiatry. 2008 Jun 30;8:51.

[74] Kobel M, Bechtel N, Specht K, et al. Structural and functional imaging approaches in attention deficit/hyperactivity disorder: does the temporal lobe play a key role? Psychiatry Res. 2010;183:230–236.

[75] Castellanos FX, Giedd JN, Marsh WL, et al. Quantitative brain magnetic resonance imaging in attention-deficit hyperactivity disorder. Arch Gen Psychiatry. 1996;53:607–616.

[76] Valera EM, Faraone SV, Murray KE, et al. Meta-analysis of structural imaging findings in attention-deficit/hyperactivity disorder. Biol Psychiatry. 2007 Jun 15;61(12):1361–9.

[77] Hair NL, Hanson JL, Wolfe BL, et al. Association of Child Poverty, Brain Development, and Academic Achievement. JAMA Pediatr. 2015 Sep;169(9):822-9.

[78] Cortese S, Kelly C, Chabernaud C, et al. Toward systems neuroscience of ADHD: a meta-analysis of 55 fMRI studies. Am J Psychiatry. 2012 Oct;169(10):1038–55.

[79] Yordanova J, Heinrich H, Kolev V, et al. Increased event-related theta activity as a psychophysiological marker of comorbidity in children with tics and attention-deficit/hyperactivity disorders. Neuroimage. 2006 Aug 15;32(2):940–55.

[80] Ogrim G, Kropotov J, Hestad K. The quantitative EEG theta/beta ratio in attention deficit/hyperactivity disorder and normal controls:

sensitivity, specificity, and behavioral correlates. Psychiatry Res. 2012 Aug 15;198(3):482–8.

[81] Snyder SM, Hall JR. A meta-analysis of quantitative EEG power associated with attention-deficit hyperactivity disorder. J Clin Neurophysiol. 2006 Oct;23(5):440–55.

[82] Mazaheri A, Fassbender C, Coffey-Corina S, et al. Differential Oscillatory Electroencephalogram Between Attention-Deficit/Hyperactivity Disorder Subtypes and Typically Developing Adolescents. Biological Psych. 2014 Sep;76(5):422–29.

[83] Lagopoulos J, Xu J, Rasmussen I, et al. Increased theta and alpha EEG activity during nondirective meditation. J Altern Complement Med. 2009 Nov;15(11):1187–92.

[84] Lomas T, Ivtzan I, Fu CH. A systematic review of the neurophysiology of mindfulness on EEG oscillations. Neurosci Biobehav Rev. 2015 Oct;57:401–10.

[85] Ilie G, Vingilis ER, Mann RE, et al. The association between traumatic brain injury and ADHD in a Canadian adult sample. J Psychiatric Res. 2015 Oct;69:174–79.

[86] Adeyemo BO, Biederman J, Zafonte R, et al. Mild traumatic brain injury and ADHD: a systematic review of the literature and meta-analysis. J Atten Disord. 2014 Oct;18(7):576–84.

[87] Biederman J, Feinberg L, Chan J, et al. Mild Traumatic Brain Injury and Attention-Deficit Hyperactivity Disorder in Young Student Athletes. J Nerv Ment Dis. 2015 Nov;203(11):813–9.

[88] Max JE, Lansing AE, Koele SL, et al. Attention deficit hyperactivity disorder in children and adolescents following traumatic brain injury. Dev Neuropsychol. 2004;25(1–2):159–77.

[89] Levin H, Hanten G, Max J, et al. Symptoms of attention-deficit/hyperactivity disorder following traumatic brain injury in children. J Dev Behav Pediatr 2007;28:108–18.

[90] Yeates KO, Armstrong K, Janusz J, et al. Long-term attention problems in children with traumatic brain injury. J Am Acad Child Adolesc Psychiatry 2005;44:574–84.

[91] Kraus MF, Susmaras T, Caughlin BP, et al. White matter integrity and cognition in chronic traumatic brain injury: a diffusion tensor imaging study. Brain. 2007 Oct;130(Pt 10):2508–19.

[92] Economidou D, Theobald DE, Robbins TW, et al. Norepinephrine and dopamine modulate impulsivity on the five-choice serial reaction time task through opponent actions in the shell and core sub-regions of the nucleus accumbens. Neuropsychopharmacology. 2012 Aug;37(9):2057–66.

[93] Volkow ND, Wang GJ, Kollins SH, et al. Evaluating dopamine reward pathway in ADHD: clinical implications. JAMA. 2009 Sep 9;302(10):1084–91.

[94] Volkow ND, Wang GJ, Newcorn JH, et al. Motivation Deficit in ADHD is Associated with Dysfunction of the Dopamine Reward Pathway. Mol Psychiatry. 2011 Nov;16(11):1147–1154.

[95] Tomasi D, Volkow ND. Functional connectivity of substantia nigra and ventral tegmental area: maturation during adolescence and effects of ADHD. Cereb Cortex. 2014 Apr;24(4):935–44.

[96] del Campo N, Fryer TD, Hong YT, et al. A positron emission tomography study of nigro-striatal dopaminergic mechanisms underlying attention: implications for ADHD and its treatment. Brain. 2013 Nov;136(Pt 11):3252–70.

[97] Maltezos S, Horder J, Coghlan S, et al. Glutamate/glutamine and neuronal integrity in adults with ADHD: a proton MRS study. Transl Psychiatry. 2014 Mar 18;4:e373.

[98] Perlov E, Philipsen A, Hesslinger B, et al. Reduced cingulate glutamate/glutamine-to-creatine ratios in adult patients with attention deficit/hyperactivity disorder–a magnet resonance spectroscopy study. J Psychiatr Res. 2007 Dec;41(11):934–41.

[99] Economidou D, Theobald DE, Robbins TW, et al. Norepinephrine and dopamine modulate impulsivity on the five-choice serial reaction time task through opponent actions in the shell and core sub-regions of the nucleus accumbens. Neuropsychopharmacology. 2012 Aug;37(9):2057–66.

[100] Volkow ND, Wang GJ, Kollins SH, et al. Evaluating dopamine reward pathway in ADHD: clinical implications. JAMA. 2009 Sep 9;302(10):1084–91.

[101] Dorval KM, Wigg KG, Crosbie J, et al. Association of the glutamate receptor subunit gene GRIN2B with attention-deficit/hyperactivity disorder. Genes Brain Behav. 2007 Jul;6(5):444–52.

[102] Elia J, Glessner JT, Wang K, et al. Genome-wide copy number variation study associates metabotropic glutamate receptor gene networks with attention deficit hyperactivity disorder. Nat Genet. 2012 Jan;44(1):78–84.

[103] Grandjean P, Landrigan PJ. Neurobehavioural effects of developmental toxicity. Lancet. 2014 Mar;13(3):330–38.

[104] Lanphear BP. The impact of toxins on the developing brain. Annu Rev Public Health. 2015 Mar 18;36:211–30.

[105] Zhang C, Xu D, Luo H, et al. Prenatal xenobiotic exposure and intrauterine hypothalamus-pituitary-adrenal axis programming alteration. Toxicology. 2014 Nov 5;325:74–84.

[106] Sherman JD. Chlorpyrifos (Dursban)-associated birth defects: report of four cases. Arch Environ Health. 1996 Jan–Feb;51(1):5–8.

[107] Unuvar T, Buyukgebiz A. Fetal and neonatal endocrine disruptors. J Clin Res Pediatr Endocrinol. 2012 Jun;4(2):51–60.

[108] Wadzinski TL, Geromini K, McKinley Brewer J, et al. Endocrine disruption in human placenta: expression of the dioxin-inducible enzyme, CYP1A1, is correlated with that of thyroid hormone-regulated genes. J Clin Endocrinol Metab. 2014 Dec;99(12):E2735–43.

[109] Giera S, Bansal R, Ortiz-Toro TM, et al. Individual polychlorinated biphenyl (PCB) congeners produce tissue- and gene-specific effects on thyroid hormone signaling during development. Endocrinology. 2011 Jul;152(7):2909–19.

[110] Pemberton HN, Franklyn JA, Kilby MD. Thyroid hormones and fetal brain development. Minerva Ginecol. 2005 Aug;57(4):367–78.

[111] de Escobar GM1, Obregón MJ, del Rey FE. Maternal thyroid hormones early in pregnancy and fetal brain development. Best Pract Res Clin Endocrinol Metab. 2004 Jun;18(2):225–48.

[112] Morreale de Escobar G1, Obregon MJ, Escobar del Rey F. Role of thyroid hormone during early brain development. Eur J Endocrinol. 2004 Nov;151 Suppl 3:U25–37.

[113] Haddow JE, Palomaki GE, Allan WC, et al. Maternal thyroid deficiency during pregnancy and subsequent neuropsychological development of the child. New Eng J Med. 1999;341:549–555.

[114] Harvard. Five numbers to remember about early childhood development. Available at: http://developingchild.harvard.edu/resources/five-numbers-to-remember-about-early-childhood-development/.

[115] Wayman GA, Yang D, Bose DD, et al. PCB-95 Promotes Dendritic Growth via Ryanodine Receptor–Dependent Mechanisms. Environ Health Persp. 2012 Jul;120(7):997-1002.

[116] Eubig PA, Aguiar A, Schantz SL. Lead and PCBs as Risk Factors for Attention Deficit/Hyperactivity Disorder. Environ Health Perspect. 2010 Dec;118(12):1654–1667.

[117] Froehlich TE, Lanphear BP, Auinger P, et al. Association of tobacco and lead exposures with attention-deficit/hyperactivity disorder. Pediatrics. 2009 Dec;124(6):e1054–63.

[118] Nigg JT, Knottnerus GM, Martel MM, et al. Low blood lead levels associated with clinically diagnosed attention-deficit/hyperactivity disorder and mediated by weak cognitive control. Biol Psychiatry. 2008 Feb 1;63(3):325–31.

[119] Wang HL, Chen XT, Yang B, et al. Case-control study of blood lead levels and attention deficit hyperactivity disorder in Chinese children. Environ Health Perspect. 2008 Oct; 116(10):1401–6.

[120] Nicolescu R, Petcu C, Cordeanu A, et al. Environmental exposure to lead, but not other neurotoxic metals, relates to core elements of ADHD in Romanian children: Performance and questionnaire data. Environmental Research. 2010;110(5):476–483.

[121] Ha M, Kwon HJ, Lim MH, et al. Low blood levels of lead and mercury and symptoms of attention deficit hyperactivity in children: a report of the children's health and environment research (CHEER). Neurotoxicology. 2009 Jan;30(1):31–6.

[122] Choi WJ1, Kwon HJ2, Lim MH, et al. Blood lead, parental marital status and the risk of attention-deficit/hyperactivity disorder in elementary school children: A longitudinal study. Psychiatry Res. 2016 Jan 6. [Epub ahead of print]

[123] Cecil KM, Brubaker CJ, Adler AM, et al. Decreased Brain Volume in Adults with Childhood Lead Exposure. PLoS Med. 2008 May;5(5):e112.

[124] Brubaker CJ, Schmithorst VJ, Haynes EN, et al. Altered myelination and axonal integrity in adults with childhood lead exposure: a diffusion tensor imaging study. Neurotoxicology. 2009 Nov;30(6):867–75.

[125] Hsieh TJ, Chuang HY, Chen YC, et al. Subclinical white matter integrity in subjects with cumulative lead exposure. Radiology. 2009 Aug;252(2):509–17.

[126] Chen YC, Yu ML, Rogan WJ, et al. A 6-year follow-up of behavior and activity disorders in the Taiwan Yu-cheng children. Am J Pub Health. 1994;84(3):415–21.

[127] Rogan WJ, Gladen BC, Hung KL, et al. Congenital poisoning by polychlorinated biphenyls and their contaminants in Taiwan. Science. 1988 Jul 15;241(4863):334–6.

[128] Jacobson JL, Jacobson SW. Dose-response in perinatal exposure to polychlorinated biphenyls (PCBs): the Michigan and North Carolina cohort studies. Toxicol Ind Health. 1996 May–Aug;12(3–4):435–45.

[129] Jacobson J, Jacobson S. Intellectual impairment in children exposed to polychlorinated biphenyls in utero. New Eng J Medicine. 1996;335:783–9.

[130] Eubig PA, Aguiar A, Schantz SL. Lead and PCBs as Risk Factors for Attention Deficit/Hyperactivity Disorder. Environ Health Perspect. 2010 Dec;118(12):1654–1667.

[131] Peper M, Klett M, Morgenstern R. Neuropsychological effects of chronic low-dose exposure to polychlorinated biphenyls (PCBs): A cross-sectional study. Environ Health. 2005;4:22.

[132] Miller VM, Kahnke T, Neu N, et al. Developmental PCB exposure induces hypothyroxinemia and sex-specific effects on cerebellum glial protein levels in rats. Int J Dev Neurosci. 2010 Nov;28(7):553–60.

[133] Brown VJ. Blocking Brain Development: How PCBs Disrupt Thyroid Hormone. Environ Health Perspect. 2005 Jul;113(7):A472–A473.

[134] Faroon O, Jones D, de Rosa C. Effects of polychlorinated biphenyls on the nervous system. Toxicol Ind Health. 2000 Sep;16(7–8):305–33.
[135] Zengin N, Yüzbaşıoğlu D, Unal F, et al. The evaluation of the genotoxicity of two food preservatives: sodium benzoate and potassium benzoate. Food Chem Toxicol. 2011 Apr;49(4):763–9.
[136] Hu M, Wang J, Cai J, et al. Analysis of Sodium Benzoate Biotoxicity using Atomic Force Microscope. Chinese J Biotechnol. 2008 Aug;24(8):1428–32.
[137] Li K, Jing Y, Yang C, et al. Increased leukemia-associated gene expression in benzene-exposed workers. Scientific Reports. 2014;4:5369.
[138] U.S. Environmental Protection Agency. Carcinogenic effects of benzene: An update. 1998 Apr.
[139] McCann D, Barrett A, Cooper A, et al. Food additives and hyperactive behaviour in 3-year-old and 8/9-year-old children in the community: a randomised, double-blinded, placebo-controlled trial. Lancet. 2007 Nov 3;370(9598):1560–7.
[140] Stevenson J, Sonuga-Barke E, McCann D, et al. The role of histamine degradation gene polymorphisms in moderating the effects of food additives on children's ADHD symptoms. Am J Psychiatry. 2010 Sep;167(9):1108–15.
[141] Committee FA, editor. Administration USFaD: Interim Toxicology Review Memorandum: Artificial Food Colors and ADHD in Childhood and Related Problem Behaviors. Washington, D.C.: Department of Health & Human Services;2011.
[142] Bouchard MF, Bellinger DC, Wright RO, et al. Attention-Deficit/Hyperactivity Disorder and Urinary Metabolites of Organophosphate Pesticides. Pediatrics. 2010 Jun;125(6):e1270–e1277.
[143] Rauh VA, Garfinkel R, Perera FP, et al. Impact of Prenatal Chlorpyrifos Exposure on Neurodevelopment in the First 3 Years of Life Among Inner-City Children. Pediatrics. 2006;118(6):e1845–59.
[144] Wagner-Schuman M, Richardson JR, Auinger P, et al. Association of pyrethroid pesticide exposure with attention-deficit/hyperactivity disorder in a nationally representative sample of U.S. children. Environ Health. 2015 May 28;14:44.
[145] Torres-Sanchez L, Schnaas L, Rothenberg SJ, et al. Prenatal p,p'-DDE exposure and neurodevelopment among children 3.5–5 years of age. Environ Health Perspect. 2013;121:263–268
[146] Boucher O, Simard MN, Muckle G, et al. Exposure to an organochlorine pesticide (chlordecone) and development of 18-month-old infants. Neurotoxicology. 2013;35:162–168

[147] Polańska K, Jurewicz J, Hanke W. Review of current evidence on the impact of pesticides, polychlorinated biphenyls and selected metals on attention deficit / hyperactivity disorder in children. Int J Occup Med Environ Health. 2013 Mar;26(1):16–38.

[148] Rubin BS. Bisphenol A: An endocrine disruptor with widespread exposure and multiple effects. J Steroid Biochem Mol Biol. 2011 Oct;127(1–2):27–34.

[149] Wenhui Qiu, Yali Zhao, Ming Yang, et al. Actions of Bisphenol A and Bisphenol S on the Reproductive Neuroendocrine System During Early Development in Zebrafish. Endocrinology. Endocrinology. 2016 Feb;157(2):636–47.

[150] Rochester JR, Bolden AL. Bisphenol S and F: A Systematic Review and Comparison of the Hormonal Activity of Bisphenol A Substitutes. Environ Health Perspect. 2015 Jul;123(7):643–50.

[151] Harley KG, Gunier RB, Kogut K, et al. Prenatal and early childhood bisphenol A concentrations and behavior in school-aged children. Environ Res. 2013 Oct;126:43–50.

[152] Evans SF, Kobrosly RW, Barrett ES, et al. Prenatal bisphenol A exposure and maternally reported behavior in boys and girls. Neurotoxicology. 2014 Dec;45:91–9.

[153] Kim BN, Cho SC, Kim Y, et al. Phthalates Exposure and Attention-Deficit/Hyperactivity Disorder in School-Age Children. Biol Psychiatry. 2009 Nov 15;66(10):958–63.

[154] Chopra V, Harley K, Lahiff, et al. Association between phthalates and attention deficit disorder and learning disability in U.S. children, 6–15 years. Environ Res. 2014 Jan;128:64–9.

[155] Malin AJ, Till C. Exposure to fluoridated water and attention deficit hyperactivity disorder prevalence among children and adolescents in the United States: an ecological association. Environ Health. 2015 Feb 27;14:17.

[156] Choi AL, Sun G, Zhang Y, et al. Developmental Fluoride Neurotoxicity: A Systematic Review and Meta-Analysis. Environ Health Perspect. 2012 Oct;120(10):1362–1368.

[157] Khan SA, et al. Relationship between dental fluorosis and intelligence quotient of school going children in and around Lucknow district: a cross-sectional study. J Clin Diagnostic Res. 2015;9(11):ZC10–15.

[158] Wasserman GA, Liu X, Parvez F, et al. Water manganese exposure and children's intellectual function in Araihazar, Bangladesh. Environ Health Perspect. 2006 Jan;114(1):124–9.

[159] Kern CH, Stanwood GD, Smith DR. Preweaning manganese exposure causes hyperactivity, disinhibition, and spatial learning and memory deficits associated with altered dopamine receptor and transporter levels. Synapse. 2010 May;64(5):363–78.

[160] Hernández-Bonilla D, Schilmann A, Montes S, et al. Environmental exposure to manganese and motor function of children in Mexico. Neurotoxicology. 2011 Oct;32(5):615–21.

[161] Amor LB, Grizenko N, Schwartz G, et al. Perinatal complications in children with attention-deficit hyperactivity disorder and their unaffected siblings. J Psychiatry Neurosci. 2005 Mar; 30(2):120–126.

[162] Milberger S, Biederman J, Faraone SV, et al. Pregnancy, delivery and infancy complications and attention deficit hyperactivity disorder: Issues of gene-environment interaction. Biol Psychiatry. 1997 Jan;41(1):65–75.

[163] Getahun D, Rhoads GG, Demissie K, et al. In Utero Exposure to Ischemic-Hypoxic Conditions and Attention-Deficit/Hyperactivity Disorder. Pediatrics. 2013 Jan;131(1):e53.

[164] Grizenko N, Fortier ME, Zadorozny C, et al. Maternal Stress during Pregnancy, ADHD Symptomatology in Children and Genotype: Gene-Environment Interaction. J Can Acad Child Adolesc Psychiatry. 2012 Feb;21(1):9–15.

[165] Grizenko N, Fortier ME, Gaudreau-Simard M, et al. The Effect of Maternal Stress during Pregnancy on IQ and ADHD Symptomatology. J Can Acad Child Adolesc Psychiatry. 2015 Fall;24(2):92–99.

[166] Silva D, Colvin L, Hagemann E, et al. Environmental Risk Factors by Gender Associated With Attention-Deficit/Hyperactivity Disorder.

[167] Cicchetti D, Rogosch F, Lynch M, et al. Resilience in maltreated children: Processes leading to adaptive outcome. Development Psychopathology. 1993;5:629–647.

[168] Deater-Deckard K, Dodge K. Externalizing behavior problems revisited: Nonlinear effects and variation by culture, context and gender. Psychological Inquiry. 1997;8:161–175

[169] Margolin G, Gordis EB. The effects of family and community violence on children. Annu Rev Psychol. 2000; 51:445–79.

[170] Anderson CA, Hinshaw SP, Simmel C. Mother-child interactions in ADHD and comparison boys: relationships with overt and covert externalizing behavior. J Abnorm Child Psychol. 1994 Apr;22(2):247–65.

[171] Braun JM, Kahn RS, Froehlich, et al. Exposures to Environmental Toxicants and Attention Deficit Hyperactivity Disorder in U.S. Children. Environ Health Perspect. 2006 Dec;114(12):1904–1909.

[172] Anastopoulos AD, Guevremont DC, Shelton TL, et al. Parenting stress among families of children with attention deficit hyperactivity disorder. J Abnorm Child Psychol. 1992 Oct;20(5):503–20.

[173] Johnston C, Mash EJ. Families of children with attention-deficit/hyperactivity disorder: review and recommendations for future research. Clin Child Fam Psychol Rev. 2001 Sep;4(3):183–207.

[174] Brown N. Associations Between Adverse Childhood Experiences and ADHD: Analysis of the 2011 National Survey of Children's Health.

[175] Becker-Blease KA, Freyd JJ. A Preliminary Study of ADHD Symptoms and Correlates: Do Abused Children Differ from Nonabused Children? J Aggression Maltreatment Trauma. 2008;17(1):133–40.

[176] Ford JD, Racusin R, Ellis CG, et al. Child maltreatment, other trauma exposure, and posttraumatic symptomatology among children with oppositional defiant and attention deficit hyperactivity disorders. Child Maltreat. 2000 Aug; 5(3):205–17.

[177] Smith AM, Hinshaw SP. Linkages Between Child Abuse and Attention-Deficit/Hyperactivity Disorder in Girls: Behavioral and Social Correlates. Child Abuse Negl. 2006 Nov; 30(11):1239–1255.

[178] Hadianfard H. Child Abuse in Group of Children with Attention Deficit-Hyperactivity Disorder in Comparison with Normal Children. Int J Community Based Nurs Midwifery. 2014 Apr;2(2):77–84.

[179] Fuller-Thomson E, Mehta R, Valeo A. Establishing a Link Between Attention Deficit Disorder/Attention Deficit Hyperactivity Disorder and Childhood Physical Abuse. J Aggression Maltreatment Trauma. 2014;23(2):188–98.

[180] Esme Fuller-Thomson, Danielle A. Lewis. The relationship between early adversities and attention-deficit/hyperactivity disorder. Child Abuse Neglect. 2015 Sep;47:94–101.

[181] Glaser D. Child abuse and neglect and the brain—A review. J Child Psychology Psychiatry. 2000 Jan;41(01):97–116.

[182] Teicher MH. The neurobiology of child abuse. Available at: http://www.theresiliencezone.com/wp-content/uploads/2015/03/Neurobiology-of-Child-Abuse.pdf.

[183] Max W, Sung HY, Shi Y. Attention deficit hyperactivity disorder among children exposed to secondhand smoke: a logistic regression analysis of secondary data. Int J Nurs Stud. 2013 Jun;50(6):797–806.

[184] Millberger S, Biederman J, Faraone SV, et al. Is maternal smoking during pregnancy a risk factor for attention deficit hyperactivity disorder in children? Am J of Psychiatry. 1996;153:1138–1142.

[185] Milberger S1, Biederman J, Faraone SV, et al. Further evidence of an association between maternal smoking during pregnancy and

attention deficit hyperactivity disorder: findings from a high-risk sample of siblings. J Clin Child Psychol. 1998 Oct;27(3):352–8.

[186] Fergusson D, Horwood L, Lynskey M. Maternal smoking before and after pregnancy: effects on behavioral outcomes in middle childhood. Pediatrics. 1993;92(6):815–22.

[187] Denson R, Nanson J, McWatters J. Hyperkinesis and maternal smoking. Can Psych Assoc J. 1975;20:183–187.

[188] Weitzman M, Gortmaker S, Sobol A. Maternal smoking and behavior problems of children. Pediatrics. 1992;90:342–349.

[189] Makin J, Fried PA, Watkinson B. A comparison of active and passive smoking during pregnancy: long-term effects. Neurotoxicology Teratology. 1991;13:5–12.

[190] Pagani LS. Environmental tobacco smoke exposure and brain development: the case of attention deficit/hyperactivity disorder. Neurosci Biobehav Rev. 2014 Jul;44:195–205.

[191] Tiesler CM1, Heinrich J. Prenatal nicotine exposure and child behavioural problems. Eur Child Adolesc Psychiatry. 2014 Oct;23(10):913–29.

[192] Ernst M, Moolchan ET, Robinson ML. Behavioral and neural consequences of prenatal exposure to nicotine. J Am Acad Child Adolesc Psychiatry. 2001 Jun;40(6):630–41.

[193] Froehlich TE, Lanphear BP, Auinger P, et al. Association of tobacco and lead exposures with attention-deficit/hyperactivity disorder. Pediatrics. 2009 Dec;124(6):e1054–63.

[194] Braun JM, Kahn RS, Froehlich T, et al. Exposures to environmental toxicants and attention deficit hyperactivity disorder in U.S. children. Environ Health Perspect. 2006 Dec;114(12):1904–9.

[195] Schober W, Szendrei K, Matzen W, et al. Use of electronic cigarettes (e-cigarettes) impairs indoor air quality and increases FeNO levels of e-cigarette consumers. Int J Hyg Environ Health. 2014 Jul;217(6):628–37.

[196] Generation Rescue. Cal-Oregon Unvaccinated Survey. Available at: http://www.generationrescue.org/resources/vaccination/cal-oregon-unvaccinated-survey/.

[197] Waly M, Olteanu H, Banerjee R, et al. Activation of methionine synthase by insulin-like growth factor-1 and dopamine: a target for neurodevelopmental toxins and thimerosal. Molecular Psychiatry. 2004;9:358–370.

[198] Brust JCM. Ethanol and Cognition: Indirect Effects, Neurotoxicity and Neuroprotection: A Review. Int J Environ Res Public Health. 2010 Apr;7(4):1540–1557.

[199] Chang LW. Neurotoxic effects of mercury—A review. Environmental Res. 1977 Dec;14(3):329-73.

[200] Josh JG. Aluminum, a neurotoxin which affects diverse metabolic reactions. Biofactors. 1990 Jul;2(3):163-9.

[201] Geier DA, Hooker BS, Kern JK, et al. A dose-response relationship between organic mercury exposure from thimerosal-containing vaccines and neurodevelopmental disorders. Int J Environ Res Public Health. 2014 Sep 5;11(9):9156-70.

[202] U.S. Food and Drug Administration. CFR – Code of Federal Regulations Title 21. Available at: http://www.accessdata.fda.gov/scripts/cdrh/cfdocs/cfcfr/cfrsearch.cfm?fr=201.323.

[203] Schultz ST, Klonoff-Cohen HS, Wingard DL, et al. Acetaminophen (paracetamol) use, measles-mumps rubella vaccination, and autistic disorder: The results of a parent survey. Autism. 2008;12(3):293–307

[204] Shaw W. Evidence that Increased Acetaminophen use in Genetically Vulnerable Children Appears to be a Major Cause of the Epidemics of Autism, Attention Deficit with Hyperactivity, and Asthma. J Restorative Med. 2013 Oct;2(1):14-29.

[205] Miranda A, Presentacion MJ. Efficacy of Cognitive-Behavioral therapy in the treatment of children with ADHD, with and without aggressiveness. Psych Schools. 2000 Mar;37(2):169–82.

[206] Carlson CL, Pelham WE, Milich R, et al. Single and combined effects of methylphenidate and behavior therapy on the classroom performance of children with attention-deficit hyperactivity disorder. J Abnormal Child Psych. 1992 Apr;20(2):213–32.

[207] Bloomquist ML, August GJ, Ostrander R. Effects of a school-based cognitive-behavioral intervention for ADHD children. J Abnormal Child Psych. 1991 Oct;19(5):591–605.

[208] Barbaresi WJ, Katusic SK, Colligan RC, et al. Long-term stimulant medication treatment of attention-deficit/hyperactivity disorder: results from a population-based study. J Dev Behav Pediatr. 2006 Feb;27(1):1–10.

[209] Barbaresi WJ, Katusic SK, Colligan RC, et al. Long-term stimulant medication treatment of attention-deficit/hyperactivity disorder: results from a population-based study. J Dev Behav Pediatr. 2014 Sep;35(7):448–57.

[210] Gottlieb S. Methylphenidate works by increasing dopamine levels. BMJ. 2001 Feb 3;322(7281):259.

[211] Kuczenski R, Segal DS. Effects of methylphenidate on extracellular dopamine, serotonin, and norepinephrine: comparison with amphetamine. J Neurochem. 1997 May;68(5):2032–7.

[212] Arnold LE. Methylphenidate vs. amphetamine: Comparative review. J Attention Disorders. 2000;3(4):200–211.

[213] Wilens TE, Adler LA, Adams J, et al. Misuse and diversion of stimulants prescribed for ADHD: a systematic review of the literature. J Am Acad Child Adolesc Psychiatry. 2008 Jan;47(1):21–31.

[214] National Institutes of Drug Abuse. DrugFacts: Stimulant ADHD Medications: Methylphenidate and Amphetamines. 2014 Jan. Available at: https://www.drugabuse.gov/publications/drugfacts/stimulant-adhd-medications-methylphenidate-amphetamines.

[215] Arria AM, O'Grady KE, Caldeira KM, et al. Nonmedical Use of Prescription Stimulants and Analgesics: Associations with Social and Academic Behaviors among College Students. J Drug Issues. 2008;38(4):1045–1060.

[216] Reske M, Eidt CA, Delis DC, et al. Non-Dependent Stimulant Users of Cocaine and Prescription Amphetamines Show Verbal Learning and Memory Deficits. Biol Psychiatry. 2010 Oct 15;68(8):762–769.

[217] Lakhan SE, Kirchgessner A. Prescription stimulants in individuals with and without attention deficit hyperactivity disorder: misuse, cognitive impact, and adverse effects. Brain Behav. 2012 Sep;2(5):661–677.

[218] Cascade E, Kalali AH, Wigal SB. Real-World Data on: Attention Deficit Hyperactivity Disorder Medication Side Effects. Psychiatry (Edgmont). 2010 Apr;7(4):13–5.

[219] Varley CK, Vincent J, Varley P, et al. Emergence of tics in children with attention deficit hyperactivity disorder treated with stimulant medications. Compr Psychiatry. 2001 May–Jun;42(3):228–33.

[220] Lipkin PH, Goldstein IJ, Adesman AR. Tics and dyskinesias associated with stimulant treatment in attention-deficit hyperactivity disorder. Arch Pediatr Adolesc Med. 1994 Aug;148(8):859–61.

[221] Martinez-Raga J, Knecht C, Szerman N, et al. Risk of serious cardiovascular problems with medications for attention-deficit hyperactivity disorder. CNS Drugs. 2013 Jan;27(1):15–30.

[222] Silva RR, Skimming JW, Muniz R. Cardiovascular safety of stimulant medications for pediatric attention-deficit hyperactivity disorder. Clin Pediatr (Phila). 2010 Sep;49(9):840–51.

[223] MacKenzie LE, Abidi S, Fisher HL, et al. Stimulant Medication and Psychotic Symptoms in Offspring of Parents With Mental Illness. Pediatrics. 2016 Jan. [Epub ahead of print]

[224] Stein M. Parental Mental Illness and Risk for Psychotic Reaction to Stimulant Drugs. Pediatrics. 2016 Jan. [Epub ahead of print]

[225] Swanson JM, Flockhart D, Udrea D, et al. Clonidine in the treatment of ADHD: questions about safety and efficacy. J Child Adolesc Psychopharmacol. 1995;5:301–04.

[226] Wilens TE, Biederman J, Geist DE, et al. Nortriptyline in the treatment of ADHD: a chart review of 58 cases. J Am Acad Child Adolesc Psychiatry. 1993 Mar;32(2):343–9.

[227] Daly JM, Wilens T. The use of tricyclic antidepressants in children and adolescents. Pediatr Clin North Am. 1998;45:1123–35.

[228] Walsh BT, Greenhill LL, Giardina EG, et al. Effects of desipramine on autonomic input to the heart. J Am Acad Child Adolesc Psychiatry. 1999 Sep;38(9):1186–92.

[229] Riddle MA, Nelson JC, Kleinman CS, et al. Sudden death in children receiving Norpramin: A review of three reported cases and commentary. J Am Acad Child Adolesc Psychiatry. 1991;30(1):104–8

[230] Faraone SV, Biederman J, Mick E. The age-dependent decline of attention deficit hyperactivity disorder: a meta-analysis of follow-up studies. Psychological Medicine. 2006;36:159–165.

[231] Kessler RC, Adler L, Barkley R, et al. The prevalence and correlates of adult ADHD in the United States: results from the national comorbidity survey replication. American Journal of Psychiatry. 2006;163:716–723.

[232] Ghanizadeh A, Haddad B. The effect of dietary education on ADHD, a randomized controlled clinical trial. Ann Gen Psychiatry. 2015 Mar 1;14:12.

[233] Park S, Cho SC, Hong YC, et al. Association between dietary behaviors and attention-deficit/hyperactivity disorder and learning disabilities in school-aged children. Psychiatry Res. 2012 Aug 15;198(3):468–76.

[234] Release Institute of Medicine (US) Committee on Military Nutrition Research; Marriott BM, editor. Food Components to Enhance Performance: An Evaluation of Potential Performance-Enhancing Food Components for Operational Rations. Washington (DC): National Academies Press (US); 1994. 13, Effects of Nutrients on Neurotransmitter Release. Available from: http://www.ncbi.nlm.nih.gov/books/NBK209058/

[235] Fernstrom JD. Large neutral amino acids: dietary effects on brain neurochemistry and function. Amino Acids. 2013 Sep;45(3):419–30.

[236] Wurtman RJ. Food consumption, neurotransmitter synthesis, and human behaviour. Experientia Suppl. 1983;44:356–69.

[237] Wolraich ML, Wilson DB, White W. The Effect of Sugar on Behavior or Cognition in Children A Meta-analysis. JAMA. 1995;274(20):1617–1621.

[238] Hoover DW, Milich R. Effects of sugar ingestion expectancies on mother-child interactions. J Abnorm Child Psychol. 1994 Aug;22(4):501–15.

[239] Schwartz DL, Gilstad-Hayden K, Carroll-Scott A, et al. Energy drinks and youth self-reported hyperactivity/inattention symptoms. Acad Pediatr. 2015 May–Jun;15(3):297–304.

[240] Lien L, Lien N, Heyerdahl S, et al. Consumption of Soft Drinks and Hyperactivity, Mental Distress, and Conduct Problems Among Adolescents in Oslo, Norway. Am J Public Health. 2006 October; 96(10):1815–1820.

[241] Kohlboeck G, Heitmueller C, Neumann C. Is there a relationship between hyperactivity/inattention symptoms and poor oral health? Results from the GINIplus and LISAplus study. Clin Oral Investig. 2013 Jan;17(5):1329–1338.

[242] Franklin JL, Mirzaei M, Wearne TA, et al. Extended exposure to caffeine and sucrose results in persistent changes to neurobiology and an age dependent response to acute methamphetamine challenge.

[243] Agrawal R, Gomez-Pinilla F. 'Metabolic syndrome' in the brain: deficiency in omega-3 fatty acid exacerbates dysfunctions in insulin receptor signalling and cognition. J Physiol. 2012;590:2485–2499.

[244] Millichap JG, Yee MM. The diet factor in attention-deficit/hyperactivity disorder. Pediatrics. 2012 Feb;129(2):330–7.

[245] Murphy JM, Pagano ME, Nachmani J, et al. The relationship of school breakfast to psychosocial and academic functioning: cross-sectional and longitudinal observations in an inner-city school sample. Arch Pediatr Adolesc Med. 1998 Sep;152(9):899–907.

[246] Basch CE. Breakfast and the achievement gap among urban minority youth. J Sch Health. 2011 Oct;81(10):635–40.

[247] Johansson J, Landgren M, Fernell E, et al. Altered tryptophan and alanine transport in fibroblasts from boys with attention-deficit/hyperactivity disorder (ADHD): an in vitro study. Behav Brain Funct. 2011;7:40.

[248] Wingen M, Kuypers KP, van de Ven V, et al. Sustained attention and serotonin: a pharmaco-fMRI study. Hum Psychopharmacol. 2008 Apr;23(3):221–30.

[249] Crockett MJ, Clark L, Robbins TW, et al. Serotonin Modulates Behavioural Reactions to Unfairness. Science. 2008 Jun 27;320(5884):1739.

[250] Rowe AH, editor. Elimination diets and the patient's allergies; a handbook of allergy. Philadelphia: Lea & Febiger; 1944.

[251] Lapage CP. Allergy, metabolism, and the autonomic nervous system. Br Med J. 1934 Dec 1;2(3856):985–7.

[252] Uhlig T, Merkenschlager A, Brandmaier R, et al. Topographic mapping of brain electrical activity in children with food-induced

attention deficit hyperkinetic disorder. Eur J Pediatr. 1997 Jul;156(7):557–61.

[253] Ferro MA, Van Lieshout RJ, Ohayon J, et al. Emotional and Behavioral Problems in Adolescents and Young Adults with Food Allergy. Allergy. 2015 Dec 30.

[254] Shanahan L, Zucker N, Copeland WE, et al. Are children and adolescents with food allergies at increased risk for psychopathology? J Psychosom Res. 2014 Dec;77(6):468–73.

[255] Arnold LE, Lofthouse N, Hurt E. Artificial food colors and attention-deficit/hyperactivity symptoms: conclusions to dye for. Neurotherapeutics. 2012 Jul;9(3):599–609.

[256] Eagle K. ADHD impacted by sulfotransferase (SULT1A) inhibition from artificial food colors and plant-based foods. Physiol Behav. 2014 Aug;135:174–9.

[257] Stevens LJ, Kuczek T, Burgess JR, et al. Dietary sensitivities and ADHD symptoms: thirty-five years of research. Clin Pediatr (Phila). 2011 Apr;50(4):279–93.

[258] Vojdani A, Vojdani C. Immune reactivity to food coloring. Altern Ther Health Med. 2015;21 Suppl 1:52–62.

[259] Stevens LJ, Kuczek T, Burgess JR, et al. Dietary sensitivities and ADHD symptoms: thirty-five years of research. Clin Pediatr (Phila). 2011 Apr;50(4):279–93.

[260] Mergenthaler P, Lindauer U, Dienel GA, et al. Sugar for the brain: the role of glucose in physiological and pathological brain function. Trends Neurosci. 2013 Oct;36(10):587–597.

[261] Blum K, Lih-Chuan Chen A, Braverman ER, et al. Attention-deficit-hyperactivity disorder and reward deficiency syndrome. Neuropsychiatr Dis Treat. 2008 Oct; 4(5):893–918.

[262] Gailliot MT, Baumeister RF. The physiology of willpower: linking blood glucose to self-control. Pers Soc Psychol Rev. 2007 Nov;11(4):303–27.

[263] McAulay V, Deary IJ, Ferguson SC, et al. Acute hypoglycemia in humans causes attentional dysfunction while nonverbal intelligence is preserved. Diabetes Care. 2001 Oct;24(10):1745–50.

[264] Ernst M, Zametkin AJ, Matochik J, et al. Intravenous dextroamphetamine and brain glucose metabolism. Neuropsychopharmacology. 1997 Dec;17(6):391–401.

[265] Kohli P, Levy BD. Resolvins and protectins: mediating solutions to inflammation. Br J Pharmacol. 2009 Oct; 158(4):960–971.

[266] Duvall MG, Levy BD. DHA- and EPA-derived resolvins, protectins, and maresins in airway inflammation. Eur J Pharmacol. 2015 Nov 3.

[267] Wu A, Ying Z, Gomez-Pinilla F. Omega-3 fatty acids supplementation restores mechanisms that maintain brain

homeostasis in traumatic brain injury. J Neurotrauma. 2007 Oct; 24(10):1587–95.

[268] Molteni R, Barnard JR, Ying Z, Roberts CK, Gomez-Pinilla F. A high-fat, refined sugar diet reduces hippocampal brain-derived neurotrophic factor, neuronal plasticity, and learning. Neuroscience. 2002;112(4):803–14.

[269] Greenwood CE, Winocur G. High-fat diets, insulin resistance and declining cognitive function. Neurobiol Aging. 2005;26 (Suppl 1):42–45

[270] Burgess JR, Stevens L, Zhang W, et al. Long-chain polyunsaturated fatty acids in children with attention-deficit hyperactivity disorder. AM J Clin Nutr. 2000;71(1):327–30.

[271] Stevens L, Zhang W, Peck L, et al. EFA supplementation in children with inattention, hyperactivity, and other disruptive behaviors. Lipids. 1996;38(10):1007–21.

[272] Richardson AJ, Puri BK. A randomized double-blind, placebo-controlled study of the effects of supplementation with highly unsaturated fatty acids on ADHD-related symptoms in children with specific learning difficulties. Prog Neuropsychopharm Biological Psych. 2002;26(2):23–39.

[273] Richardson AJ, Puri BK. A randomized double-blind, placebo-controlled study of the effects of supplementation with highly unsaturated fatty acids on ADHD-related symptoms in children with specific learning difficulties. Prog Neuropsychopharm Biological Psych. 2002;26(2):23–39.

[274] Voigt RG, Llorente AM, Jeensen CL, et al. A randomized, double-blind, placebo-controlled trial of docosahexaenoic acid supplementation in children with attention-deficit/hyperactivity disorder. J Pediatrics. 2001;139(2):189–96.

[275] Sinn N. Nutritional and dietary influences on attention deficit hyperactivity disorder. Nutr Rev. 2008 Oct;66(10):558–68.

[276] Burdge GC, Jones AE, Wootton SA. Eicosapentaenoic acids are the principal products of alpha-linolenic acid metabolism in young men. Br J Nutr. 2002;88(4):355–64.

[277] Burdge GC, Wootton SA. Conversion of alpha-linolenic acid to eicosapentaenoic, docosapentaenoic and docosahexaenoic in young women. Br J Nutr. 2002;88(4):411–20.

[278] Zheng JS, Hu XJ, Zhao YM, et al. Intake of fish and marine n-3 polyunsaturated fatty acids and risk of breast cancer: meta-analysis of data from 21 independent prospective cohort studies. BMJ. 2013 June;346:f3706.

[279] Harris W, Pottala J, Sands S, et al. Comparison of the effects of fish and fish-oil capsules on the n-3 fatty acid content of blood cells

and plasma phospholipids. Am J Clin Nutr. 2007 Dec;86(6):1621–1625.

[280] Konikowska K, Regulska-Ilow B, Rózańska D. The influence of components of diet on the symptoms of ADHD in children. Rocz Panstw Zakl Hig. 2012;63(2):127–34.

[281] Millchap JG, Yee MM. The Diet Factor in Attention-Deficit/Hyperactivity Disorder. 2012 Feb;129(2):330–37.

[282] Pinera DJ, Connor JR. Iron in the Brain: An Important Contributor in Normal and Diseased States. 2000 Dec;6(6):435–53.

[283] Youdim MB. Brain iron deficiency and excess; cognitive impairment and neurodegeneration with involvement of striatum and hippocampus. Neurotox Res. 2008 Aug;14(1):45–56.

[284] Jahanshad N, Kohannim O, Hibar DP, et al. Brain structure in healthy adults is related to serum transferrin and the H63D polymorphism in the HFE gene. PNAS. 2012;109(14):E851–59.

[285] Halterman JS, Kaczorowski JM, Aligne CA, et al. Iron deficiency and cognitive achievement among school-aged children and adolescents in the United States. Pediatrics. 2001;107(6):1381–86.

[286] Takeda A. Zinc homeostasis and functions of zinc in the brain. Biometals. 2001 Sep–Dec;14(3–4):343–51.

[287] Rink L, Gabriel P. Zinc and the immune system. Proc Nutr Soc. 2000;59:541–552.

[288] Pan E, Zhang XA, Huang Z, et al. Vesicular Zinc Promotes Presynaptic and Inhibits Postsynaptic Long-Term Potentiation of Mossy Fiber-CA3 Synapse. Neuron. 2011;71(6):1116.

[289] Bettger WJ, Reeves PG, Moscatelli EA, et al. Interaction of zinc and essential fatty acids in the rat. J Nutr. 1979;109:480–88.

[290] Arnold LE, DiSilvestro RA. Zinc in attentiondeficit/hyperactivity disorder. J Child Adolesc Psychopharmacol. 2005;15(4):619–627.

[291] Pfeiffer CC, Braverman ER. Zinc, the brain and behavior. Biol Psychiatry. 1982 Apr;17(4):513–32.

[292] Liu J. Raine A, Venables PH, et al. Malnutrition at Age 3 Years and Externalizing Behavior Problems at Ages 8, 11, and 17 Years. Am J Psychiatry. 2004 Nov; 161(11):2005–2013.

[293] Arnold LE, DiSilvestro RA. Zinc in attentiondeficit/hyperactivity disorder. J Child Adolesc Psychopharmacol. 2005;15(4):619–627

[294] Slutsky I, Abumaria N, Wu LJ, et al. Enhancement of learning and memory by elevating brain magnesium. Neuron. 2010 Jan 28;65(2):165–77.

[295] Bush AI. Kalzium ist nicht alles. Neuron. 2010 Jan 28;65(2):143–4.

[296] Slutsky I, Sadeghpour S, Li B, et al. Enhancement of synaptic plasticity through chronically reduced Ca2+ flux during uncorrelated activity. Neuron. 2004 Dec 2;44(5):835–49.

[297] Scassellati C, Bonvicini C, Faraone SV, et al. Review: Biomarkers and AttentionDeficit/Hyperactivity Disorder: A Systematic Review and Meta-Analyses. J Am Acad Child Adolesc Psychiatry. 2012;51:1003–1019.

[298] Kozielec T, Starobrat-Hermelin B. Assessment of magnesium levels in children with attention deficit hyperactivity disorder (ADHD). Magnes Res. 1997 Jun;10(2):143–8.

[299] El Blaza F, Ahmed AlShahawi H, Zahra S, et al. Magnesium supplementation in children with attention deficit hyperactivity disorder. Egyptian J Med Human Genetics. 2016 Jan;17(1):63–70.

[300] Hossein-nezhad A, Spira A, Holick MF. Influence of vitamin D status and vitamin D3 supplementation on genome wide expression of white blood cells: a randomized double-blind clinical trial. PLoS One. 2013;8(3):e58725.

[301] Hossein-nezhad A, Spira A, Holick MF. Influence of vitamin D status and vitamin D3 supplementation on genome wide expression of white blood cells: a randomized double-blind clinical trial. PLoS One. 2013;8(3):e58725.

[302] Soni M, Kos K, Lang IA, et al. Vitamin D and cognitive function. Scand J Clin Lab Invest Suppl. 2012;243:79–82.

[303] Eyles DW, Smith S, Kinobe R, et al. Distribution of the Vitamin D receptor and 1α-hydroxylase in human brain. J Chem Neuroanat. 2005;29:21–30.

[304] Ellison-Wright I, Ellison-Wright Z, Bullmore E. Structural brain change in Attention Deficit Hyperactivity Disorder identified by meta-analysis. BMC Psychiatry. 2008;8:51.

[305] Goksgur SB, Tufan AE, Semiz M, et al. Vitamin D status in children with attention-deficit–hyperactivity disorder. Pediatrics Int. 2014 Aug;56(4):515–19.

[306] Amieva MR, Vogelmann R, Covacci A, et al. Disruption of the epithelial apical-junctional complex by Helicobacter pylori CagA. Science. 2003;300:1430–1434.

[307] Thanabalasuriar A, Koutsouris A, Weflen A, et al. The bacterial virulence factor NleA is required for the disruption of intestinal tight junctions by enteropathogenic Escherichia coli. Cell Microbiol. 2010;12:31–41.

[308] Boyle EC, Brown NF, Finlay BB. Salmonella enterica serovar Typhimurium effectors SopB, SopE, SopE2 and SipA disrupt tight junction structure and function. Cell Microbiol. 2006;8:1946–1957.

[309] Rosenfeldt V, Benfeldt E, Valerius NH, et al. Effect of probiotics on gastrointestinal symptoms and small intestinal permeability in children with atopic dermatitis. J Pediatr. 2004;145:612–616.

[310] Madsen K, Cornish A, Soper P, et al. Probiotic bacteria enhance murine and human intestinal epithelial barrier function. Gastroenterology. 2001;121:580–591.
[311] Stratiki Z, Costalos C, Sevastiadou S, et al. The effect of a bifidobacterium supplemented bovine milk on intestinal permeability of preterm infants. Early Hum Dev. 2007;83:575–579.
[312] Heijtz RD, Wang S, Anuar F, et al. Normal gut microbiota modulates brain development and behavior. PNAS. 2011 Feb;3(1):e00261–11.
[313] Bercik P, Park AJ, Sinclair D, et al. The anxiolytic effect of Bifidobacterium longum NCC3001 involves vagal pathways for gut-brain communication. Neurogastroenterol Motil. 2011 Dec;23(12):1132–9.
[314] Bravo JA, Forsythe P, Chew MV, et al. Ingestion of Lactobacillus strain regulates emotional behavior and central GABA receptor expression in a mouse via the vagus nerve. Proc Natl Acad Sci U S A. 2011 Sep 20;108(38):16050–5.
[315] Ochoa-Repáraz J, Kasper LH. The Second Brain: Is the Gut Microbiota a Link Between Obesity and Central Nervous System Disorders? Curr Obes Rep. 2016 Feb 11. [Epub ahead of print]
[316] Indrio F, Mauro A, Riezzo G, et al. Prophylactic use of probiotic in the prevention of colic, regurgitation, and functional constipation. A randomized clinical trial. JAMA Pediatr. 2014;168(3):228–33.
[317] Chau K, Lau E2, Greenberg S, et al. Probiotics for infantile colic: a randomized, double-blind, placebo-controlled trial investigating Lactobacillus reuteri DSM 17938. J Pediatr. 2015 Jan;166(1):74–8.
[318] Videhult FK, West CE. Nutrition, gut microbiota and child health outcomes. Curr Opin Clin Nutr Metab Care. 2016 Feb 11. [Epub ahead of print]
[319] Onubi OJ, Poobalan AS, Dineen B, et al. Effects of probiotics on child growth: a systematic review. J Health Popul Nutr. 2015 May 2;34(1):8.
[320] Hansen CH, Nielsen DS, Kverka M, et al. Patterns of early gut colonization shape future immune responses of the host. PLoS One. 2012;7(3):e34043.
[321] Goulet O. Potential role of the intestinal microbiota in programming health and disease. Nutr Rev. 2015 Aug;73 Suppl 1:32–40.
[322] Vitetta L, Briskey D, Alford H, et al. Probiotics, prebiotics and the gastrointestinal tract in health and disease. Inflammopharmacology. 2014 Jun;22(3):135–54.
[323] Martin R, Nauta AJ, Ben Amor K, et al. Early life: gut microbiota and immune development in infancy. Benef Microbes. 2010 Nov;1(4):367–82.

[324] Gomez, et al. Gut microbiome of coexisting BaAka pygmies and Bantu reflects gradients of traditional subsistence patterns. Cell Reports. 2016 Feb. [Epub ahead of print]

[325] Logan AC, Jacka FN, Prescott SL. Immune-Microbiota Interactions: Dysbiosis as a Global Health Issue. Curr Allergy Asthma Rep. 2016 Jan;16(2):13.

[326] Carabotti M, Scirocco A, Maselli MA, et al. The gut-brain axis: interactions between enteric microbiota, central and enteric nervous systems. Ann Gastroenterol. 2015 Apr–Jun;28(2):203–209.

[327] Vitetta L, Coulson S, Linnane AW, et al. The Gastrointestinal Microbiome and Musculoskeletal Diseases: A Beneficial Role for Probiotics and Prebiotics. Pathogens. 2013 Dec;2(4):606–626.

[328] Ettinger G, MacDonald K, Reid G, et al. The influence of the human microbiome and probiotics on cardiovascular health. Gut Microbes. 2014 5(6):719–28.

[329] Kelly D, King T, Aminov R. Importance of microbial colonization of the gut in early life to the development of immunity. Mutat Res. 2007 Sep 1;622(1–2):58–69.

[330] Tlaskalová-Hogenová H, Stepánková R, Hudcovic T, et al. Commensal bacteria (normal microflora), mucosal immunity and chronic inflammatory and autoimmune diseases. Immunol Lett. 2004 May 15;93(2–3):97–108.

[331] Goulet O. Potential role of the intestinal microbiota in programming health and disease. Nutr Rev. 2015 Aug;73 Suppl 1:32–40.

[332] Mahler GJ, Esch MB, Glahn RP, et al. Characterization of a gastrointestinal tract microscale cell culture analog used to predict drug toxicity. Biotechnol Bioeng. 2009 Sep 1;104(1):193–205.

[333] Carding S, Verbeke K, Vipond DT, et al. Dysbiosis of the gut microbiota in disease. Microbial Ecol Health Dis. 2015;26:26191.

[334] Partty A, Kalliomaki M, Wacklin P, et al. A possible link between early probiotic intervention and the risk of neuropsychiatric disorders later in childhood: a randomized trial. Pediatr Res. 2015 Jun;77(6):823–8.

[335] Perkin GD, Murray-Lyon I. Neurology and the gastrointestinal system. J Neurol Neurosurg Psychiatry. 1998;65:291–300.

[336] Dietrich W1, Erbguth F. [Neurological complications of inflammatory intestinal diseases]. Fortschr Neurol Psychiatr. 2003 Aug;71(8):406–14.

[337] Consumer Reports Magazine: July 2011. Available at: http://www.consumerreports.org/cro/magazine-archive/2011/july/food/yogurt/overview/index.htm.

[338] Beganović J, Pavunc AL, Gjuračić K, et al. Improved sauerkraut production with probiotic strain Lactobacillus plantarum L4 and

Leuconostoc mesenteroides LMG 7954. J Food Sci. 2011 Mar;76(2):M124–9.

[339] Altay F, Karbancıoglu-Güler F, Daskaya-Dikmen C. A review on traditional Turkish fermented non-alcoholic beverages: microbiota, fermentation process and quality characteristics. Int J Food Microbiol. 2013 Oct;167(1):44–56.

[340] Rea MC, et al. Irish Kefir like grains: their structure, microbial composition and fermentation kinetics. J Appl Bacteriology. 1996;81(1):83–94.

[341] Birch EE, Garfield S, Castaneda Y, et al. Visual acuity and cognitive outcomes at 4 years of age in a double-blind, randomized trial of long-chain polyunsaturated fatty acid-supplemented infant formula. Early Hum Dev. 2007 May;83(5):279–84.

[342] Willatts P, Forsyth JS, DiModugno MK, Varma S, Colvin M. Effect of long-chain polyunsaturated fatty acids in infant formula on problem solving at 10 months of age. Lancet. 1998 Aug 29;352(9129):688–91.

[343] Chang CY, Ke DS, Chen JY. Essential fatty acids and human brain. Acta Neurol Taiwan. 2009 Dec;18(4):231–41.

[344] Martinez M. Tissue levels of polyunsaturated fatty acids during early human development. J Pediatr. 1992;120(4 Pt 2):S129–S138.

[345] Kohlboeck G, Glaser C, Tiesler C, et al. Effect of fatty acid status in cord blood serum on children's behavioral difficulties at 10 y of age: results from the LISAplus Study. Am J Clin Nutr. 2011 Dec;94(6):1592–9.

[346] Singh M. Essential fatty acids, DHA and human brain. Indian J Pediatr. 2005 Mar;72(3):239–42.

[347] Helland IB, Smith L, Saarem K, et al. Maternal supplementation with very-long-chain n-3 fatty acids during pregnancy and lactation augments children's IQ at 4 years of age. Pediatrics. 2003 Jan;111(1):e39–44.

[348] Auestad N, Halter R, Hall RT, et al. Growth and development in term infants fed long-chain polyunsaturated fatty acids: A double-masked, randomized, parallel, prospective, multivariate study. Pediatrics. 2001;108(2):372–381.

[349] Helland IB, Smith L, Saarem K, et al. Maternal supplementation with very-long-chain n-3 fatty acids during pregnancy and lactation augments children's IQ at 4 years of age. Pediatrics. 2003 Jan;111(1):e39–e44.

[350] Strickland AD. Prevention of cerebral palsy, autism spectrum disorder, and attention deficit-hyperactivity disorder. Med Hypotheses. 2014 May;82(5):522–8.

351 Craft D. Essential Fatty Acids & The Brain. Available at: http://www.diannecraft.org/essential-fatty-acids-the-brain/.
352 McNamara RK, Able J, Jandacek R, et al. Docosahexaenoic acid supplementation increases prefrontal cortex activation during sustained attention in healthy boys: a placebo-controlled, dose-ranging, functional magnetic resonance imaging study. Am J Clin Nutr. 2010 Apr;91(4):1060–7.
353 Bradbury J. Docosahexaenoic Acid (DHA): An Ancient Nutrient for the Modern Human Brain. Nutrients. 2011 May;3(5):529–554.
354 Broadhurst CL, Wang Y, Crawford MA, et al. Brain-specific lipids from marine, lacustrine, or terrestrial food resources: potential impact on early African Homo sapiens. Comp Biochem Physiol B Biochem Mol Biol. 2002 Apr;131(4):653–73.
355 Tan ZS, Harris WS, Beiser AS, et al. Red blood cell omega-3 fatty acid levels and markers of accelerated brain aging. Neurology. 2012 Feb 28;78(9):658–64.
356 Pottala JV, Yaffe K, Robinson JG, et al. Higher RBC EPA + DHA corresponds with larger total brain and hippocampal volumes: WHIMS-MRI study. Neurology. 2014 Feb 4;82(5):435–42.
357 Crippa A, Agostoni C, Mauri M, et al. Polyunsaturated Fatty Acids Are Associated With Behavior But Not With Cognition in Children With and Without ADHD: An Italian study. J Atten Disord. 2016 Feb 9. [Epub ahead of print]
358 Gow RV, Vallee-Tourangeau F, Crawford MA, et al. Omega-3 fatty acids are inversely related to callous and unemotional traits in adolescent boys with attention deficit hyperactivity disorder. Prostaglandins Leukot Essent Fatty Acids. 2013 Jun;88(6):411–8.
359 Antalis CJ, Stevens LJ, Campbell M, et al. Omega-3 fatty acid status in attention-deficit/hyperactivity disorder. Prostaglandins Leukot Essent Fatty Acids. 2006;75:299–308.
360 Transler C, Eilander A, Mitchell S, et al. The impact of polyunsaturated fatty acids in reducing child attention deficit and hyperactivity disorders. J Atten Disord. 2010;14:232–246.
361 Bos DJ, Oranje B, Veerhoek ES, et al. Reduced Symptoms of Inattention after Dietary Omega-3 Fatty Acid Supplementation in Boys with and without Attention Deficit/Hyperactivity Disorder. Neuropsychopharmacology. 2015 Sep;40(10):2298–306.
362 Milte CM, Parletta N, Buckley JD, et al. Increased Erythrocyte Eicosapentaenoic Acid and Docosahexaenoic Acid Are Associated With Improved Attention and Behavior in Children With ADHD in a Randomized Controlled Three-Way Crossover Trial. J Atten Disord. 2015 Nov;19(11):954–64.
363 Hariri M, Djazayery A, Djalali M, et al. Effect of n-3 supplementation on hyperactivity, oxidative stress and inflammatory

mediators in children with attention-deficit-hyperactivity disorder. Malays J Nutr. 2012 Dec;18(3):329–35.

[364] Hirayama S, Hamazaki T, Terasawa K. Effect of docosahexaenoic acid-containing food administration on symptoms of attention-deficit/hyperactivity disorder - a placebo-controlled double-blind study. Eur J Clin Nutr. 2004 Mar;58(3):467–73.

[365] Voigt RG, Llorente AM, Jensen CL, et al. A randomized, double-blind, placebo-controlled trial of docosahexaenoic acid supplementation in children with attention-deficit/hyperactivity disorder. J Pediatr. 2001 Aug;139(2):189–96.

[366] Milte CM, Parletta N, Buckley JD, et al. Eicosapentaenoic and docosahexaenoic acids, cognition, and behavior in children with attention-deficit/hyperactivity disorder: a randomized controlled trial. Nutrition. 2012 Jun;28(6):670–7.

[367] Laidlaw M, Cokerline CA, Rowe WJ. A randomized clinical trial to determine the efficacy of manufacturers' recommended doses of omega-3 fatty acids from different sources in facilitating cardiovascular disease risk reduction. Lipids Health Dis. 2014 Jun 21;13:99.

[368] Kris-Etherton PM, Taylor DS, Yu-Poth S, et al. Polyunsaturated fatty acids in the food chain in the United States. Am J Clin Nutr. 2000 Jan;71(1 Suppl):179S–88S.

[369] Kapoor R, Huang YS. Gamma linolenic acid: an antiinflammatory omega-6 fatty acid. Curr Pharm Biotechnol. 2006 Dec;7(6):531–4.

[370] Tate G, Mandell BF, Laposata M, et al. Suppression of acute and chronic inflammation by dietary gamma linolenic acid. J Rheumatol. 1989 Jun;16(6):729–34.

[371] Aman MG, Mitchell EA, Turbott SH. The effects of essential fatty acid supplementation by Efamol in hyperactive children. J Abnorm Child Psychol. 1987 Mar;15(1):75–90.

[372] Grassman V, Santos-Galduroz RF, Fernandez Galduroz JC. Effects of Low Doses of Polyunsaturated Fatty Acids on the Attention Deficit/Hyperactivity Disorder of Children: A Systematic Review. Curr Neuropharmacol. 2013 Mar;11(2):186–196.

[373] Johnson M, Ostlund S, Fransson G, et al. Omega-3/omega-6 fatty acids for attention deficit hyperactivity disorder: a randomized placebo-controlled trial in children and adolescents. J Atten Disord. 2009;12(5):394–401.

[374] Eyles DW, Burne TH, McGrath JJ. Vitamin D, effects on brain development, adult brain function and the links between low levels of vitamin D and neuropsychiatric disease. Front Neuroendocrinol. 2013;34(1):47–64.

[375] Humble MB, Gustafsson S, Bejerot S. Low serum levels of 25-hydroxyvitamin D (25-OHD) among psychiatric out-patients in

Sweden: relations with season, age, ethnic origin and psychiatric diagnosis. J Steroid Biochem Mol Biol. 2010;121(1-2):467–70.

[376] Patrick RP, Ames BN. Vitamin D and the omega-3 fatty acids control serotonin synthesis and action, part 2: relevance for ADHD, bipolar disorder, schizophrenia, and impulsive behavior. FASEB J. 2015 Jun;29(6):2207–22.

[377] Sharif MR, Madani M, Tabatabaei F, et al. The Relationship between Serum Vitamin D Level and Attention Deficit Hyperactivity Disorder. Iran J Child Neurol. 2015 Fall;9(4):48–53.

[378] Shang-Guan LL, Zhao YR. [Serum levels of 25-hydroxyvitamin D in children with attention deficit hyperactivity disorder]. Zhongguo Dang Dai Er Ke Za Zhi. 2015 Aug;17(8):837–40.

[379] Forrest KY, Stuhldreher WL. Prevalence and correlates of vitamin D deficiency in US adults. Nutr Res. 2011 Jan;31(1):48–54.

[380] Chen TC, Chimeh F, Lu Z, et al. Factors that influence the cutaneous synthesis and dietary sources of vitamin D. Arch Biochem Biophys. 2007;460:213–7.

[381] Clemens TL, Adams JS, Henderson SL, Holick MF. Increased skin pigment reduces the capacity of skin to synthesise vitamin D3. Lancet. 1982;74–76.

[382] Fuleihan GEH, Nabulsi M, Choucair M, et al. Hypovitaminosis D in healthy schoolchildren. Pediatrics. 2001;107:53–9.

[383] Sedrani SH. Low 25-hydroxyvitamin D and normal serum calcium concentrations in Saudi Arabia: Riyadh region. Ann Nutr Metab. 1984;28:181–5.

[384] Tangpricha V, Pearce EN, Chen TC, et al. Vitamin D insufficiency among free-living healthy young adults. Am J Med. 2002;112:659–62.

[385] Gordon CM, DePeter KC, Estherann G, et al. Prevalence of vitamin D deficiency among healthy adolescents. Arch Pediatr Adolesc Med. 2004;158:531–7.

[386] Marwaha RK, Tandon N, Reddy D, et al. Vitamin D and bone mineral density status of healthy schoolchildren in northern India. Am J Clin Nutr. 2005;82:477–82.

[387] McGrath JJ, Kimlin MG, Saha S, et al. Vitamin D insufficiency in south-east Queensland. Med J Aust. 2001;174:150–1.

[388] Kechrid Z, Hamdi M, Naziroğlu M, et al. Vitamin D supplementation modulates blood and tissue zinc, liver glutathione and blood biochemical parameters in diabetic rats on a zinc-deficient diet. Biol Trace Elem Res. 2012 Sep;148(3):371–7.

[389] Garcion E, Wion-Barbot N, Montero-Menei CN, et al. New clues about vitamin D functions in the nervous system. Trends Endocrinol Metab. 2002;13(3):100–5.

[390] Garcion E, Thanh XD, Bled F, et al. 1,25-dihydroxy vitamin D3 regulates gamma-glutamyl transpeptidase activity in rat brain. Neurosci Lett. 1996 Oct 4;216(3):183–6.

[391] Sears ME. Chelation: harnessing and enhancing heavy metal detoxification–a review. ScientificWorldJournal. 2013 Apr 18;2013:219840.

[392] James SJ, Slikker W 3rd, Melnyk S, et al. Thimerosal neurotoxicity is associated with glutathione depletion: protection with glutathione precursors. Neurotoxicology. 2005 Jan;26(1):1–8.

[393] Garcion E, Wion-Barbot N, Montero-Menei CN, et al. New clues about vitamin D functions in the nervous system. Trends Endocrinol Metab. 2002;13(3):100–5.

[394] Dringen R, Hirrlinger J. Glutathione pathways in the brain. Biol Chem. 2003 Apr;384(4):505–16.

[395] Dringen R, Gutterer JM, Hirrlinger J. Glutathione metabolism in brain metabolic interaction between astrocytes and neurons in the defense against reactive oxygen species. Eur J Biochem. 2000 Aug;267(16):4912–6.

[396] Ruchi K, Anil Kumar S, Sunil G, et al. Antioxidant activity in children with ADHD – a comparison in untreated and treated subjects with normal children. Int Med J Malaysia. 2011 Jun;10(1):31–35.

[397] Morales E, Julvez J, Torrent M, et al. Vitamin D in Pregnancy and Attention Deficit Hyperactivity Disorder-like Symptoms in Childhood. Epidemiology. 2015 Jul;26(4):458–65.

[398] Maalouf J, Nabulsi M, Vieth R, et al. Short- and Long-Term Safety of Weekly High-Dose Vitamin D3 Supplementation in School Children. J Clin Endocrinol Metab. 2008 Jul;93(7):2693–701.

[399] Cashman KD. Vitamin D in childhood and adolescence. Postgrad Med J. 2007 Apr; 83(978):230–235.

[400] Bener A, Kamal M, Bener H, et al. Higher prevalence of iron deficiency as strong predictor of attention deficit hyperactivity disorder in children. Ann Med Health Sci Res. 2014 Sep;4(Suppl 3):S291–7.

[401] Lepping P, Huber M. Role of zinc in the pathogenesis of attention-deficit hyperactivity disorder: implications for research and treatment. CNS Drugs. 2010 Sep;24(9):721–8.

[402] Dodig-Curković K, Dovhanj J, Curković M, et al. [The role of zinc in the treatment of hyperactivity disorder in children]. Acta Med Croatica. 2009 Oct;63(4):307–13.

[403] Arnold LE, DiSilvestro RA. Zinc in attention-deficit/hyperactivity disorder. J Child Adolesc Psychopharmacol. 2005 Aug;15(4):619–27.

[404] Chen MH, Su TP, Chen YS, et al. Association between psychiatric disorders and iron deficiency anemia among children and adolescents: a nationwide population-based study. BMC Psychiatry. 2013 Jun 4;13:161.

[405] Arnold LE, Disilvestro RA, Bozzolo D, et al. Zinc for attention-deficit/hyperactivity disorder: placebo-controlled double-blind pilot trial alone and combined with amphetamine. J Child Adolesc Psychopharmacol. 2011 Feb;21(1):1–19.

[406] Calarge C, Farmer C, DiSilvestro R, et al. Serum ferritin and amphetamine response in youth with attention-deficit/hyperactivity disorder. J Child Adolesc Psychopharmacol. 2010 Dec;20(6):495–502.

[407] Arnold LE, Bozzolo H, Hollway J, et al. Serum zinc correlates with parent- and teacher-rated inattention in children with attention-deficit/hyperactivity disorder. J Child Adolesc Psychopharmacol. 2005 Aug;15(4):628–36.

[408] DiGirolamo AM, Ramirez-Zea M, Wang M, et al. Randomized trial of the effect of zinc supplementation on the mental health of school-age children in Guatemala. Am J Clin Nutr. 2010 Nov;92(5):1241–50.

[409] Zamora J, Velásquez A, Troncoso L, et al. [Zinc in the therapy of the attention-deficit/hyperactivity disorder in children. A preliminary randomized controlled trial]. Arch Latinoam Nutr. 2011 Sep;61(3):242–6.

[410] Akhondzadeh S, Mohammadi MR, Khademi M. Zinc sulfate as an adjunct to methylphenidate for the treatment of attention deficit hyperactivity disorder in children: a double blind and randomized trial [ISRCTN64132371]. BMC Psychiatry. 2004 Apr 8;4:9.

[411] Uçkardeş Y, Ozmert EN, Unal F, et al. Effects of zinc supplementation on parent and teacher behaviour rating scores in low socioeconomic level Turkish primary school children. Acta Paediatr. 2009 Apr;98(4):731–6.

[412] Bilici M, Yildirim F, Kandil S, et al. Double-blind, placebo-controlled study of zinc sulfate in the treatment of attention deficit hyperactivity disorder. Prog Neuropsychopharmacol Biol Psychiatry. 2004 Jan;28(1):181–90.

[413] Oner O, Oner P, Bozkurt OH, et al. Effects of zinc and ferritin levels on parent and teacher reported symptom scores in attention deficit hyperactivity disorder. Child Psychiatry Hum Dev. 2010 Aug;41(4):441–7.

[414] Calarge CA, Murry DJ, Ziegler EE, et al. Serum Ferritin, Weight Gain, Disruptive Behavior, and Extrapyramidal Symptoms in Risperidone-Treated Youth. J Child Adolesc Psychopharmacol. 2016 Feb 19. [Epub ahead of print]

415 Oner P, Oner O, Azik FM, et al. Ferritin and hyperactivity ratings in attention deficit hyperactivity disorder. Pediatr Int. 2012 Oct;54(5):688–92.

416 Abou-Khadra MK, Amin OR, Shaker OG, et al. Parent-reported sleep problems, symptom ratings, and serum ferritin levels in children with attention-deficit/hyperactivity disorder: a case control study. BMC Pediatr. 2013 Dec 30;13:217.

417 Merino-Andreu M. [Attention deficit hyperactivity disorder and restless legs syndrome in children]. Rev Neurol. 2011 Mar 1;52 Suppl 1:S85–95.

418 Frenette E. Restless legs syndrome in children: a review and update on pharmacological options. Curr Pharm Des. 2011;17(15):1436–42.

419 Soto-Insuga V, Calleja ML, Prados M, et al. [Role of iron in the treatment of attention deficit-hyperactivity disorder]. An Pediatr (Barc). 2013 Oct;79(4):230–5.

420 Sever Y, Ashkenazi A, Tyano S, et al. Iron treatment in children with attention deficit hyperactivity disorder. A preliminary report. Neuropsychobiology. 1997;35:178–80.

421 Slutsky I, Abumaria N, Wu LJ, et al. Enhancement of learning and memory by elevating brain magnesium. Neuron. 2010 Jan 28;65(2):165–77.

422 Slutsky I, Abumaria N, Wu LJ, et al. Enhancement of learning and memory by elevating brain magnesium. Neuron. 2010 Jan 28;65(2):165–77.

423 McKee JA, Brewer RP, Macy GE, et al. Analysis of the brain bioavailability of peripherally administered magnesium sulfate: A study in humans with acute brain injury undergoing prolonged induced hypermagnesemia. Crit Care Med. 2005 Mar;33(3):661–6.

424 Li W, Yu J, Liu Y, et al. Elevation of brain magnesium prevents synaptic loss and reverses cognitive deficits in Alzheimer's disease mouse model. Mol Brain. 2014 Sep 13;7:65.

425 Slutsky I, Abumaria N, Wu LJ, et al. Enhancement of learning and memory by elevating brain magnesium. Neuron. 2010 Jan 28;65(2):165–77.

426 Slutsky I, Abumaria N, Wu LJ, et al. Enhancement of learning and memory by elevating brain magnesium. Neuron. 2010 Jan 28;65(2):165–77.

427 Jia S1, Liu Y1, Shi Y, et al. Magnesium Supplementation Potentiates Neural Stem Cell Proliferation in the Hippocampus of Young and Aged Mice. J Cell Physiol. 2016 Jan 11.

428 Kornblum HI. Stem Cells and Stroke Recovery: Introduction. Stroke. 2007;38:810–816

[429] Slutsky I, Abumaria N, Wu LJ, et al. Enhancement of learning and memory by elevating brain magnesium. Neuron. 2010 Jan 28;65(2):165–77.

[430] Scassellati C, Bonvicini C, Faraone SV, et al. Biomarkers and attentiondeficit/hyperactivity disorder: a systematic review and meta-analyses. Journal of the American Academy of Child and Adolescent Psychiatry. 2012 Oct;51(10):1003–1019.

[431] Irmisch G, Thome J, Reis O, et al. Modified magnesium and lipoproteins in children with attention deficit hyperactivity disorder (ADHD). The world journal of biological psychiatry: the official journal of the World Federation of Societies of Biological Psychiatry. 2011 Sep;12(Suppl 1):63–65.

[432] Antalis CJ, Stevens LJ, Campbell M, et al. Omega-3 fatty acid status in attention-deficit/hyperactivity disorder. Prostaglandins, leukotrienes, and essential fatty acids. 2006 Oct–Nov;75(4–5):299–308.

[433] Nogovitsina OR, Levitina EV. [Effect of MAGNE-B6 on the clinical and biochemical manifestations of the syndrome of attention deficit and hyperactivity in children]. Eksp Klin Farmakol. 2006 Jan–Feb;69(1):74–7.

[434] Mousain-Bosc M, Roche M, Rapin J, et al. Magnesium VitB6 intake reduces central nervous system hyperexcitability in children. J Am Coll Nutr. 2004 Oct;23(5):545S–548S.

[435] Schmidt ME, Kruesi MJ, Elia J, et al. Effect of dextroamphetamine and methylphenidate on calcium and magnesium concentration in hyperactive boys. Psychiatry research. 1994 Nov;54(2):199–210.

[436] Mousain-Bosc M, Roche M, Polge A, et al. Improvement of neurobehavioral disorders in children supplemented with magnesium-vitamin B6. I. Attention deficit hyperactivity disorders. Magnes Res. 2006 Mar;19(1):46–52.

[437] Arnold LE, Hurt E, Lofthouse N. Attention-deficit/hyperactivity disorder: dietary and nutritional treatments. Child Adolesc Psychiatr Clin N Am. 2013 Jul;22(3):381–402, v.

[438] Food and Nutrition Board, Institute of Medicine. Dietary Reference Intakes for Calcium, Phosphorus, Magnesium, Vitamin D, and Fluoride. Washington, DC: National Academy Press, 1999. Available at: http://books.nap.edu/books/0309063507/html/index.html.

[439] Birrer RB, Shallash AJ, Totten V. Hypermagnesemia-induced fatality following epsom salt gargles. J Emerg Med. 2002;22:185–8.

[440] Institute of Medicine (IOM). Food and Nutrition Board. Dietary Reference Intakes: Calcium, Phosphorus, Magnesium, Vitamin D and Fluoride. Washington, DC: National Academy Press, 1997.

[441] Institute of Medicine. Food and Nutrition Board. Dietary Reference Intakes: Thiamin, Riboflavin, Niacin, Vitamin B6, Folate, Vitamin B12, Pantothenic Acid, Biotin, and Choline. Washington, DC: National Academy Press; 1998.

[442] Luzzi R, Belcaro G, Zulli C, et al. Pycnogenol® supplementation improves cognitive function, attention and mental performance in students. Panminerva Med. 2011 Sep;53(3 Suppl 1):75–82.

[443] Belcaro G, Luzzi R, Dugall M, et al. Pycnogenol® improves cognitive function, attention, mental performance and specific professional skills in healthy professionals aged 35–55. J Neurosurg Sci. 2014 Dec;58(4):239–48. [Epub 2014 Mar 28]

[444] Uttara B, Singh AV, Zamboni P, et al. Oxidative Stress and Neurodegenerative Diseases: A Review of Upstream and Downstream Antioxidant Therapeutic Options. Curr Neuropharmacol. 2009 Mar;7(1):65–74.

[445] Belcaro G, Dugall M, Ippolito E, et al. The COFU3 Study. Improvement in cognitive function, attention, mental performance with Pycnogenol® in healthy subjects (55–70) with high oxidative stress. J Neurosci. 2015 Dec;59(4):437–46.

[446] Sarris J, Kean J, Schweitzer I, et al. Complementary medicines (herbal and nutritional products) in the treatment of Attention Deficit Hyperactivity Disorder (ADHD): a systematic review of the evidence. Complement Ther Med. 2011 Aug;19(4):216–27.

[447] Trebatická J, Kopasová S, Hradecná Z, et al. Treatment of ADHD with French maritime pine bark extract, Pycnogenol. Eur Child Adolesc Psychiatry. 2006 Sep;15(6):329–35.

[448] Dvoráková M, Sivonová M, Trebatická J, et al. The effect of polyphenolic extract from pine bark, Pycnogenol, on the level of glutathione in children suffering from attention deficit hyperactivity disorder (ADHD). Redox Rep. 2006;11(4):163–72.

[449] Chovanová Z, Muchová J, Sivonová M, et al. Effect of polyphenolic extract, Pycnogenol, on the level of 8-oxoguanine in children suffering from attention deficit/hyperactivity disorder. Free Radic Res. 2006 Sep;40(9):1003–10.

[450] Dvoráková M, Jezová D, Blazícek P, et al. Urinary catecholamines in children with attention deficit hyperactivity disorder (ADHD): modulation by a polyphenolic extract from pine bark (pycnogenol). Nutr Neurosci. 2007 Jun–Aug;10(3–4):151–7.

[451] Hirayama S, Terasawa K, Rabeler R, et al. The effect of phosphatidylserine administration on memory and symptoms of attention-deficit hyperactivity disorder: a randomised, double-blind, placebo-controlled clinical trial. J Hum Nutr Diet. 2014 Apr;27 Suppl 2:284–91.

[452] Manor I, Magen A, Keidar D, et al. The effect of phosphatidylserine containing Omega 3 fatty-acids on attention-deficit hyperactivity disorder symptoms in children: A double-blind placebo-controlled trial, followed by an open-label extension. Eur Psych. 2012 Jul;27(5):335–42.

[453] Vaisman N, Kaysar N, Zaruk-Adasha Y, et al. Correlation between changes in blood fatty acid composition and visual sustained attention performance in children with inattention: effect of dietary n-3 fatty acids containing phospholipids. Am J Clin Nutr 2008;87:1170–80.

[454] Kidd PM. Attention deficit/hyperactivity disorder (ADHD) in children: rationale for its integrative management. Altern Med Rev. 2000 Oct;5(5):402–28.

[455] Oyama Y, Chikahisa L, Ueha T, et al. Ginkgo biloba extract protects brain neurons against oxidative stress induced by hydrogen peroxide. Brain Res. 1996 Mar 18;712(2):349–52.

[456] Wei T, Ni Y, Hou J, et al. Hydrogen peroxide-induced oxidative damage and apoptosis in cerebellar granule cells: protection by Ginkgo biloba extract. Pharmacol Res. 2000 Apr;41(4):427–33.

[457] Kleijnen J, Knipschild P. Ginkgo biloba for cerebral insufficiency. Br J Clin Pharmacol. 1992 Oct;34(4):352–8.

[458] Ahlemeyer B, Krieglstein J. Neuroprotective effects of Ginkgo biloba extract. Cell Mol Life Sci. 2003 Sep;60(9):1779–92.

[459] Fehske CJ, Leuner K, Müller WE. Ginkgo biloba extract (EGb761) influences monoaminergic neurotransmission via inhibition of NE uptake, but not MAO activity after chronic treatment. Pharmacol Res. 2009 Jul;60(1):68–73.

[460] Wang J, Chen W, Wang Y. A ginkgo biloba extract promotes proliferation of endogenous neural stem cells in vascular dementia rats. Neural Regen Res. 2013 Jun 25;8(18):1655–1662.

[461] Sun L, Zhuang W, Xu X, et al. The effect of injection of EGb 761 into the lateral ventricle on hippocampal cell apoptosis and stem cell stimulation in situ of the ischemic/reperfusion rat model. Neurosci Lett. 2013 Oct 25;555:123–8.

[462] Kepp O, Menger L, Vacchelli E, et al. Anticancer activity of cardiac glycosides: At the frontier between cell-autonomous and immunological effects. Oncoimmunology. 2012 Dec 1; 1(9):1640–1642.

[463] Dong X, Zheng L, Lu S, et al. Neuroprotective effects of pretreatment of ginsenoside Rb1 on severe cerebral ischemia-induced injuries in aged mice: Involvement of anti-oxidant signaling. Geriatr Gerontol Int. 2015 Dec 29. [Epub ahead of print]

[464] Nabavi SF, Sureda A, Habtemariam S, et al. Ginsenoside Rd and ischemic stroke; a short review of literatures. J Ginseng Res. 2015 Oct;39(4):299–303.

[465] Wang CZ, Anderson S, DU W, et al. Red ginseng and cancer treatment. Chin J Nat Med. 2016 Jan;14(1):7–16.

[466] Yeo HB, Yoon HK, Lee HJ, et al. Effects of Korean Red Ginseng on Cognitive and Motor Function: A Double-blind, Randomized, Placebo-controlled Trial. J Ginseng Res. 2012 Apr;36(2):190–197.

[467] Scholey A, Ossoukhova A, Owen L, et al. Effects of American ginseng (Panax quinquefolius) on neurocognitive function: an acute, randomised, double-blind, placebo-controlled, crossover study. Psychopharmacology (Berl). 2010 Oct;212(3):345–356.

[468] D'Angelo L, Grimaldi R, Caravaggi M, et al. A double-blind, placebo-controlled clinical study on the effect of a standardized ginseng extract on psychomotor performance in healthy volunteers. J Ethnopharmacol. 1986 Apr–May;16(1):15–22.

[469] Niederhofer H. Panax ginseng may improve some symptoms of attention-deficit hyperactivity disorder. J Diet Suppl. 2009;6(1):22–7.

[470] Lyon MR, Cline JC, Totosy de Zepetnek J, et al. Effect of the herbal extract combination Panax quinquefolium and Ginkgo biloba on attention-deficit hyperactivity disorder: a pilot study. J Psychiatry Neurosci. 2001 May;26(3):221–8.

[471] Nam Y, Shin EJ, Shin SW, et al. YY162 prevents ADHD-like behavioral side effects and cytotoxicity induced by Aroclor1254 via interactive signaling between antioxidant potential, BDNF/TrkB, DAT and NET. Food Chem Toxicol. 2014 Mar;65:280–92.

[472] Niederhofer H. Panax ginseng may improve some symptoms of attention-deficit hyperactivity disorder. J Diet Suppl. 2009;6(1):22–7.

[473] Lee SH, Park WS, Lim MH. Clinical effects of Korean red ginseng on attention deficit hyperactivity disorder in children: an observational study. J Ginseng Res. 2011 Jun;35(2):226–34.

[474] Ko HJ, Kim I, Kim JB, et al. Effects of Korean red ginseng extract on behavior in children with symptoms of inattention and hyperactivity/impulsivity: a double-blind randomized placebo-controlled trial. J Child Adolesc Psychopharmacol. 2014 Nov;24(9):501–8.

[475] Niederhofer H. Ginkgo biloba treating patients with attention-deficit disorder. Phytother Res. 2010 Jan;24(1):26–7.

[476] Salehi B, Imani R, Mohammadi MR, et al. Ginkgo biloba for attention-deficit/hyperactivity disorder in children and adolescents: a double blind, randomized controlled trial. Prog Neuropsychopharmacol Biol Psychiatry. 2010 Feb 1;34(1):76–80.

[477] Shakibaei F, Radmanesh M, Salari E, et al. Ginkgo biloba in the treatment of attention-deficit/hyperactivity disorder in children and adolescents. A randomized, placebo-controlled, trial. Complement Ther Clin Pract. 2015 May;21(2):61–7.

[478] Uebel-von Sandersleben H, Rothenberger A, Albrecht B, et al. Ginkgo biloba extract EGb 761® in children with ADHD. Z Kinder Jugendpsychiatr Psychother. 2014 Sep;42(5):337–47.

[479] Kako H, Fukumoto S, Kobayashi Y, et al. Effects of direct exposure of green odour components on dopamine release from rat brain striatal slices and PC12 cells. Brain Res Bull. 2008 Mar;75(5):706–12.

[480] Komiya M, Takeuchi T, Harada E. Lemon oil vapor causes an antistress effect via modulating the 5-HT and DA activities in mice. Behav Brain Res. 2006 Sep;172(2):240–49.

[481] Chioca LR, Ferro MM, Baretta IP, et al. Anxiolytic-like effect of lavender essential oil inhalation in mice: participation of serotonergic but not GABBAA/benzodiazepine neurotransmission. J Ethnopharmacol. 2013 May;147(2):412–18.

[482] L M Lopes C, Goncalves e Sa C, de Almeida AA, et al. Sedative anxiolytic and antidepressant activities of Citrus limon (Burn) essential oil in mice. Pharmazie. 2011 Aug;66(8):623–27.

[483] Kiecolt-Glaser JK, Graham JE, Malarkey WB, et al. Olfactory influences on mood and autonomic, endocrine, and immune function. Psychoneuroendocrinology. 2008 Apr;33(3):328–39.

[484] Niederhofer H. Observational study: Matricaria chamomilla may improve some symptoms of attention-deficit hyperactivity disorder. Phytomedicine. 2009 Apr;16(4):284–86.

[485] Matsubara E, Fukagawa M, Okmoto T, et al. Volatiles emitted from the leaves of Laurus nobilis L. improve vigilance performance in visual discrimination task. Biomed Res. 2011 Feb;32(1):19–28.

[486] Barker S, Grayhem P, Koon J, et al. Improved performance on clerical tasks associated with administration of peppermint odor. Percept Mot Skills. 2003 Dec;97(3 Pt 1):1007–10.

[487] Matsubara E, Shimizu K, Fukagawa M, et al. Volatiles emitted from the roots of Vetiveria zizanioides suppress the decline in attention during a visual display terminal task. Biomed Res. 2012;33(5):299–308.

[488] Murali R, Karthikeyan A, Saravanan R. Protective effects of D-limonene on lipid peroxidation and antioxidant enzymes in streptozotocin-induced diabetic rats. Basic Clin Pharmacol Toxicol. 2013 Mar;112(3):175–81.

[489] Chaudhary SC, Siddiqui MS, Athar M, et al. D-limonene modulates inflammation, oxidative stress and Ras-ERK pathway to

inhibit murine skin tumorigenesis. Hum Exp Toxicol. 2012 Aug;31(8):799–811.

[490] Fukumoto S, Sawasaki E, Okuyama S, et al. Flavor components of monoterpenes in citrus essential oils enhance the release of monoamines from rat brain slices. Nutr Neurosci. 2006 Feb–Apr;9(1–2):73–80.

[491] Vaajoki A, Kankkunen P, Pietilä AM, et al. Music as a nursing intervention: effects of music listening on blood pressure, heart rate, and respiratory rate in abdominal surgery patients. Nurs Health Sci. 2011 Dec;13(4):412–8.

[492] Siritunga S, Wijewardena K, Ekanayaka R, et al. Effect of music on blood pressure, pulse rate and respiratory rate of asymptomatic individuals: A randomized controlled trial. Health. 2013;5(4A):59–64.

[493] Beck SL. The therapeutic use of music for cancer-related pain. Oncology Nursing Forum. 1991;18:1327–37.

[494] Tan X, Yowler CJ, Super DM, et al. The efficacy of music therapy protocols for decreasing pain, anxiety, and muscle tension levels during burn dressing changes: a prospective randomized crossover trial. J Burn Care Res. 2010 Jul–Aug;31(4):590–7.

[495] Akbas A, Gulpinar MT, Sancak EB, et al. The effect of music therapy during shockwave lithotripsy on patient relaxation, anxiety, and pain perception. Ren Fail. 2016 Feb;38(1):46–9.

[496] Seither-Preisler A, Parncutt R, Schneider P, et al. Size and synchronization of auditory cortex promotes musical, literacy, and attentional skills in children. J Neurosci. 2014 Aug 13;34(33):10937–49.

[497] Krick CM, Argstatter H. Neural correlates of the Heidelberg Music Therapy: indicators for the regeneration of auditory cortex in tinnitus patients? Neural Regen Res. 2015 Sep;10(9):1373–1375.

[498] Okamoto H, Stracke H, Stoll W, et al. Listening to tailor-made notched music reduces tinnitus loudness and tinnitus-related auditory cortex activity. Proc Natl Acad Sci U S A. 2010 Jan 19;107(3):1207–10.

[499] Salimpoor VN, Benovoy M, Larcher K, et al. Anatomically distinct dopamine release during anticipation and experience of peak emotion to music. Nature Neuroscience. 2011;14:257–62.

[500] Nguyen A. Using Classical Music to Increase Productivity in Elementary School Students with Attention Deficit Hyperactivity Disorder. Available at: http://scholarscompass.vcu.edu/cgi/viewcontent.cgi?article=1056&context=uresposters.

[501] Rothmann K, Hillmer JM, Hosser D, et al. [Evaluation of the Musical Concentration Training with Pepe (MusiKo mit Pepe) for

children with attention deficits]. Z Kinder Jugendpsychiatrie Psychother. 2014 Sep;42(5):325–35.

[502] Rickson DJ. Instructional and improvisational models of music therapy with adolescents who have attention deficit hyperactivity disorder (ADHD): a comparison of the effects on motor impulsivity. J Music Ther. 2006 Spring;43(1):39–62.

[503] Kanduri C, Raijas P, Ahvenainen M, et al. The effect of listening to music on human transcriptome. PeerJ. 2015;3:e830

[504] Koenig K, Kinnealey M. Comparative Outcomes of Children with ADHD: Treatment Versus Delayed Treatment Control Condition, presented May 13, 2005 at the 2005 American Occupational Therapy Association Meeting.

[505] Lee HS, Song CS. Effects of therapeutic climbing activities wearing a weighted vest on a child with attention deficit hyperactivity disorder: a case study. J Phys Ther Sci. 2015 Oct;27(10):3337–9.

[506] Wilkes S, Cordier R, Bundy A, et al. A play-based intervention for children with ADHD: a pilot study. Aust Occup Ther J. 2011 Aug;58(4):231–40.

[507] Wilkes-Gillan S, Bundy A, Cordier R, et al. Eighteen-month follow-up of a play-based intervention to improve the social play skills of children with attention deficit hyperactivity disorder. Aust Occup Ther J. 2014 Oct;61(5):299–307.

[508] Reynolds F. Occupational Therapy for Children with Attention Deficit Hyperactivity Disorder (ADHD), Part 2: A Multicentre Evaluation of an Assessment and Treatment Package. Br J Occupational Ther. 2007 Oct;70(10):440–48.

ABOUT THE AUTHOR

Dr. Scott A. Johnson is the bestselling author of ten books and more than 300 articles featured in online and print publications. He is the creator and founder of the Integrative Essential Oils Essential Oil Certification Program, and the originator of the Waterfall Technique®. He has a doctorate in naturopathy, is a board-certified alternative medical practitioner (AMP), Certified Elite Essential Oil Specialist (CEEOS), Certified Clinical Master Aromatherapist (CCMA), and Certified Professional Coach (CPC). His evidence-based approach to natural healing and experience conducting medical research make him one of the world's leading experts on the therapeutic application of essential oils. Dr. Johnson pioneered evidence-based essential oil therapy, which combines the art of ancient healing with modern science to maximize the benefits of essential oils. One of his research focuses is the safety of essential oils, and he has published internationally on the subject. He is an acclaimed international speaker and has delivered keynote presentations across North America, Europe, and Asia. Dr. Johnson draws on his wealth of experience and diverse educational background as he travels the globe to share the secrets of natural healing with those who seek greater wellness.

Connect with Dr. Johnson

Twitter: @DocScottJohnson

Facebook: /AuthorScottAJohnson

Website: authorscott.com

INDEX

A
Abuse, child, 18, 43-44, 78
abuse, medication, 63, 64, 66
acetylcholine, 87, 117
Adderall, 61, 62
administrators, school, 14, 15, 18,
    71, 72, 76, 78, 79, 137
AGEs, 82
allergies, food, 81, 85-86
ALA, 63, 89, 90
alpha waves, 29, 30, 31
American Academy of
    Pediatrics, 51, 58, 108
American Medical
    Association, 13
amino acids, 82, 84, 87, 88
anxiety, 18, 29, 30, 43, 64, 65, 68
    69, 83, 110, 112, 114,
    123, 124, 125
Aplenzin, 68
aspartate, 87
atomoxetine hydrochloride, 66
ATP, 88
axon, 25, 31

B
bacteria, 95, 97
basal ganglia, 8, 26, 42
behavior therapy, 12, 51, 52-54,
    60, 79, 137
behaviors, risky, 10
Benzedrine, 8
beta waves, 29, 30, 120, 125
bipolar disorder, 18
birth, complications, 42-43
blood-brain barrier, 46, 117
BPA, 36, 40
brainwaves, 28, 30, 31
breakfast, 56, 83
Budeprion, 68
Buproban, 68

C
caffeine, 83, 115
carbohydrates, refined, 56, 81,
    82, 85,89, 90, 138
central nervous system, 25, 26,
    32, 34, 47, 61, 62, 96,
    98, 112, 124
cerebellum, 8, 23, 26, 27
child abuse and neglect, 18, 43-
    44, 78
chlorpyrifos, 36, 39
cigarettes, 45
circadian rhythm, 12, 13, 18, 55
classical conditioning, 52
classical music, 57, 131, 132,
    135, 138
clonidine hydrochloride, 66
cocaine, 61
communication, neuronal, 26, 48,
    91, 108, 117, 125
compliance, medication, 69, 70
Concerta, 61
copy number variants, 22, 23
corpus callosum, 27
cortex maturation, 25

D
DAT1 (SLC6A3), 21
Daytrana, 61
delta waves, 28, 29, 92
density, synaptic, 92
depression, 8, 18, 64, 65, 66, 68,
    69, 83, 110, 123, 124
desipramine hydrochloride, 67
Desoxyn, 62
Dexedrine, 61
dextromethylphenidate
    hydrochloride, 62
Dextrostat, 61
DHA, 89, 90, 91, 101-106, 107,
    117, 118, 121
dioxins, 105

L

Lapage, CP, 85
lead, 33, 36, 37, 38, 41
lisdexamfetamine dimesylate, 62
liver, 34, 68, 69, 88, 108

M

magnesium, 92-93, 106, 109,
    111-114, 122
magnesium-L-threonate, 112,
    113, 114, 122
manganese, 36, 41-42, 109
marital problems, 10
marketing, 10-11, 12, 18
medication,
    discontinuance, 69-70
meditation, 23, 29, 31
mental illness, 14
mercury, 46, 47
Metadate, 61
methamphetamine
    hydrochloride, 62
methylphenidate, 8, 61, 62, 120
microbial, 95, 96
middle frontal gyrus, 26, 30
mood, 9, 21, 28, 55, 64, 68, 70,
    92, 110, 114, 117, 122,
    123
music therapy, 129-132
myelin, 25, 26, 35, 37, 87, 91

N

neuron, 21, 23, 25, 26, 28, 32,
    33, 35, 36, 47, 48, 84,
    87, 90, 91, 93, 107, 108,
    112, 116, 117, 119, 120,
    125
nontricyclic antidepressant, 67
nonstimulants, 60, 61, 65-69
noradrenaline, 32, 33, 61 ,62,
    63, 66, 67, 68, 82 ,84,
    87, 116, 119, 123, 124,
    125

norepinephrine, 32, 33, 61 ,62,
    63, 66, 67, 68, 82 ,84,
    87, 116, 119, 123, 124,
    125
Norpramin, 67, 69
nortriptyline hydrochloride, 67
nutrition, 23, 81-100, 101, 137

O

occipitoparietal, 26
occupational therapy, 129,
    132-135, 136
omega-3 fatty acids, 89-91, 92,
    101, 102
operant conditioning, 52
organophosphates, 36, 39
oxidative stress, 48, 104, 108,
    115, 116, 119, 120

P

Pamelor, 67, 68
parenting, 9, 54, 55
parents, 12, 39, 43, 48, 51, 54,
    55, 56, 58, 60, 63, 69,
    70, 71, 72, 73, 74, 76,
    78, 79, 81, 82, 87, 90,
    100, 101, 104, 105, 106,
    110, 111, 130, 133, 136
PBDEs, 37
performance-enhancing
    drugs, 15, 64
pesticides, 36, 39-40,
phosphatidylserine, 116-118
phthalates, 41, 47
plasticity, 90, 92, 135
polymorphisms, 21, 32, 39
positive reinforcement, 54
positron emission
    tomography, 88
prefrontal cortex, 8, 24, 37, 93
pregnancy, 35, 40 ,41, 42, 43, 45,
    91, 101, 102, 103, 105,
    106, 108, 121
preservatives, food, 36, 38-39,

V

vagus nerve, 99
vestibular, 134
vitamin D, 93-94, 106-108, 122
Vyvanse, 62, 63

W

Wellbutrin, 67, 69
white matter, 25, 26, 31, 35,
        37, 91
withholding privileges, 53, 54
World Health
        Organization, 15, 40

Z

zinc, 91-92, 106, 109-110, 122
Zyban, 68